ADVANCED STATISTICS

ADVANCED STATISTICS

with applications
to physical education

H. HARRISON CLARKE
University of Oregon

DAVID H. CLARKE
University of Maryland

Prentice-Hall, Inc., Englewood Cliffs, New Jersey

ISBN: 0-13-013847-9

Library of Congress Catalog Card Number: 73-149970

10   9   8   7   6   5   4   3   2   1

PRINTED IN THE UNITED STATES OF AMERICA

Prentice-Hall International, Inc., *London*
Prentice-Hall of Australia, Pty. Ltd., *Sydney*
Prentice-Hall of Canada, Ltd., *Toronto*
Prentice-Hall of India Private Limited, *New Delhi*
Prentice-Hall of Japan, Inc., *Tokyo*

To our alma mater,
Springfield College,
where it all began

CONTENTS

APPENDIX TABLES

PREFACE

This textbook continues the statistics material in our book, *Research Processes in Physical Education, Recreation, and Health* (Englewood Cliffs, N. J.: Prentice-Hall, Inc., 1970) by carrying the presentation into advanced statistics. The amount of statistics covered is sufficient for a second course on this subject. The main topics are one-way and two-way analysis of variance with post hoc tests of significance, analysis of covariance applied to pretest means and pretest covariates, partial and multiple correlations, prediction in deviation, score, and standard score forms, Wherry-Doolittle method of multiple correlation and prediction, special correlational methods, and nonparametric statistics.

The statistical methods presented in *Research Processes* start with the most elementary aspects of frequency-table construction and continue through two-variable correlation. These materials are sufficient for a beginning, or first course, in statistics. The chapters are: 7. Tabulation, Central Tendency, Percentiles; 8. Measures of Variability; 9. The Normal Curve; 10. Reliability and Tests of Significance; and 11. Product-Moment Correlation.

Although *Advanced Statistics* was written with the research needs of the physical educator in mind, its applications may be readily extended to psychology and all fields of education. The statistics are the same as those used in these other areas. The illustrations are drawn from physical and motor growth and development and from physical education problems. The researcher in another field may simply substitute his own test data in the problems presented.

Every effort has been made to make advanced statistics as simple as possible. The need for advanced mathematical background has been minimized. The derivations of the various formulae have not been shown; rather, the computations are described, basic assumptions are explained, and applications to research data are made.

The authors wish to acknowledge the assistance of John M. Montgomery, Graduate Research Assistant, University of Oregon, for his assistance in checking the accuracy of the computations for many of the problems contained in this book. Mr. Montgomery is now in the Department of Kinesiology, Simon Fraser University, Burnaby, British Columbia, Canada.

ADVANCED STATISTICS

ANALYSIS
OF
VARIANCE

Need for Analysis of Variance

Analysis of variance is an extension of the study of the significance of differences between means. The use of the t ratio for this purpose was presented in Chapter 10 of *Research Processes*.[1] This method is proper when the difference between the means of two samples is tested. However, when more than two samples are involved the following complications arise:

    1. If several sample means are to be compared, each with all the others, the investigator could pair off all combinations and compute the t ratio for the difference between each pair. The number of t ratios would be the same as the number of games in round-robin play, as indicated by the formula: $N(N - 1)/2$. Thus, if five sample means are involved, the number of t ratios by the pairing method is 10; for ten samples, the number is 45. By analysis of variance, an overall test of significance is made between any number of sample means. An F ratio is derived which indicates whether or not any significant differences exist.

    2. The t ratio is appropriate as a test of significance when two independent sample means are compared. In this instance, the t test and the analysis of variance test are equivalent. The F ratio obtained from analysis of variance with two sample means is the square of t: $F = t^2$, or $t = \sqrt{F}$. When more than two groups are compared, the means are no longer completely independent, as each sample is serving more than once in the significance tests. For example, with four samples, A, B, C, and D, the comparisons would be:

---

[1] In this text, reference to *Research Processes* is to Clarke and Clarke, *Research Processes in Physical Education, Recreation, and Health* (Englewood Cliffs, N.J.: Prentice-Hall, Inc., 1970).

A vs B   B vs C
A vs C   B vs D
A vs D   C vs D

Each single sample is represented not just once but three times in the tests of significance, rather than utilizing three independent samples. Analysis of variance compensates for this situation and is the proper test of significance to use under this circumstance.

3. Further, if many differences between sample means were tested for significance by pairs utilizing the *t* ratio, 5 per cent and 1 per cent would be expected to reach the .05 and .01 levels of significance respectively. A simultaneous test of significance resolves this issue; analysis of variance indicates whether or not differences within the whole distribution of sample means could have occurred by chance.

4. Finally, if each pair of sample means is tested separately for a significant difference, the estimate of population variance is limited to the two samples involved. In analysis of variance, the null hypothesis is applied to all the samples, i.e., the data from all samples can be used in estimating the population variance. Thus, greater stability in the variance estimate is realized. In order to adopt this practice, however, the variances of the separate samples must be reasonably comparable.

In the paragraphs above, reference is made to one-way analysis of variance. In this instance, individual scores for each sample are arranged in parallel columns with means and variances computed for each. Analysis of variance can also be extended to multiple-way processes. In two-way analysis, two factors or treatments operate together. In this instance, three *F* ratios are computed, one each for the columns, the rows, and interaction. To illustrate: Badgley[2] studied the effects on ankle flexibility of various conditions for administering whirlpool baths. Four water temperatures and four lengths of time in the water were systematically varied. The range of motion of the ankle joint was measured before and after each bath; the difference between these tests indicated the treatment effect. The three *F* tests were for differences in water temperature, length of time in the water, and combinations of temperature and time (interaction).

Standard Deviation of Combined Samples

So that the reader may gain some initial familiarity with the terms and concepts of analysis of variance, the discussion will begin with an explanation of the process of obtaining the standard deviation of combined samples from

[2] Marion E. Badgley, "A Study of the Effect of the Whirlpool Bath on Range of Motion of the Right Ankle under Selected Conditions," Master's Thesis, University of Oregon, 1957.

the standard deviations of separate samples. In this explanation, the Σx^2, also known as the sum of squares (SS), will provide the basis for the computation. As will be recognized, SS is the essential element in the standard deviation formula: $\sigma = \sqrt{\Sigma x^2 / N}$. Given the following three sets (A, B, and C) and the combined or total (T):

	A	B	C	T
N	20	25	30	75
M	10.0	12.0	12.5	11.7
SS	80.0	132.5	189.0	480.0
σ^2	4.0	5.3	6.3	6.4
σ	2.0	2.3	2.5	2.53

The standard deviation of 2.53 for the combined sets (T) cannot be obtained by averaging the standard deviations of the three sets. This average is: $(2.0 + 2.3 + 2.5)/3 = 2.27$. Furthermore, it cannot be obtained by computing a weighted mean of the set standard deviations. Thus:

$$[(20 \times 2.0) + (25 \times 2.3) + 30 \times 2.5)] \div 75 = 2.27$$

If the set means were all the same, the weighted average of the standard deviations would equal the standard deviation of the combined groups. This result emphasizes the fact that standard deviations are obtained as squared deviations from their respective means. And, a most important concept in analysis of variance, two sources of variance exist: the variance *within sets* and the varince *between sets*.

By taking both variances into account, the standard deviation of the combined groups can be determined through computation of SS for the total. The formula is:

$$\Sigma x_t^2 = \Sigma x_a^2 + \Sigma x_b^2 + \Sigma x_c^2 + n_a d_a^2 + n_b d_b^2 + n_c d_c^2 \qquad (1.1)$$

in which:

Σx_t^2 = sum of squared deviations of all scores from total mean

$\Sigma x_a^2, \Sigma x_b^2, \Sigma x_c^2$ = sum of squared deviations of set scores from their respective means

n_a, n_b, n_c = number of scores in separate set distributions

d_a, d_b, d_c = deviations of separate set means from total mean

Thus, for this problem (formula 1.1):

$$\Sigma x_t^2 = 80.0 + 132.5 + 189.0 + 20(10 - 11.7)^2 + 25(12 - 11.7)^2 \\ + 30(12.5 - 11.7)^2$$

$$= 80.0 + 132.5 + 189.0 + 57.8 + 2.3 + 19.2$$
$$= 480.8$$

To complete for standard deviation:

$$\sigma^2 = \Sigma x_t^2/N = 480.8/75 = 6.4$$
$$\sigma = \sqrt{6.4} = 2.53$$

We should note that the small n refers to the set number and the large N to the total number for the problem. Formula 1.1 can be expanded or repressed to accommodate any number of sets.

In this illustration, Σx_a^2, Σx_b^2, Σx_c^2 provide the within-sets variance for the various sets. The deviations are from the means of each subsample. The between-sets variance is obtained from d_a, d_b, d_c, deviations of the set means from the total mean. In effect, the differences between means are being compared indirectly through their variances from a common mean, M_t. Thus, the total sum of squares is made up of two components: the within-sets and the between-sets variances. In an analysis of variance problem, the F ratio is derived as a ratio between these variances.

One-Way Analysis of Variance

The computation of one-way analysis of variance is comparable to the procedures described above for obtaining the standard deviation of the combined sets from the separate sets of scores. These sets are designated as k; if three sets are involved, as in the standard deviation problem, $k = 3$.

MEAN SQUARES

To obtain the F ratio, however, the mean sum of squares must be obtained for each of the within-sets and between-sets variances; these variances are designated as $(MS)_w$ and $(MS)_b$ respectively. To obtain the mean squares, the two sums of squares are divided by their respective degrees of freedom (df); one df is lost in computing each mean. To illustrate, assume k sets of n scores. For example, $k = 5$; $n = 10$; $N = 50$:

Within Sets. Five sets are involved; thus five df are lost, one for each set. The degrees of freedom may be expressed in two ways:

$$(df)_w = N - k = 50 - 5 = 45$$

or,

$$= k(n - 1) = 5(10 - 1) = 45$$

Therefore:

$$(MS)_w = \frac{(SS)w}{k(n-1)} = \frac{\Sigma x_s^2}{k(n-1)} = \frac{\Sigma x_s^2}{N-k} \qquad (1.2)$$

Note: The small s in these formulas refer to computations within the separate sets.

Between Sets.   As the between-sets variance is obtained by relating the several set means to the total mean, one df is lost from the number of set means. Thus:

$$(df)_b = k - 1 = 5 - 1 = 4$$

Therefore:

$$(MS)_b = \frac{(SS)_b}{k-1} = \frac{n\Sigma d^2}{k-1} \qquad (1.3)$$

The use of $n\Sigma d^2$ is appropriate in the formula when the number of scores in each set is the same, as is true in this illustration ($n = 10$). Since the problem to be illustrated next also has a constant n, this formula will be applied to it.

Problem Solution

The data for this one-way analysis problem consist of the skeletal ages and weights of 12-year-old boys. Three maturity groups, advanced, normal, and retarded, were formed based on their skeletal ages. As related to a much larger number of boys, the advanced and retarded boys had skeletal ages one standard deviation above and below the mean respectively; the skeletal ages of the normal group were within $\pm.5$ standard deviation from the mean. The body weights of the three sets thus formed appear in Table 1-1. In this problem, then, $k = 3$, $n = 10$, and $N = 30$. The steps in making the computations follow; reference is made to the parts of Table 1-1.

1. *Part A:* Compute the sums and the means of sets 1, 2, and 3 and of the total scores of all sets combined (ΣX_t and M_t). As can be seen at the bottom of part A of the table, the set means are 140.7, 98.3, and 76.9 pounds; the total mean is 105.3 pounds. It is the differences between these set means that will be tested for significance by analysis of variance.

2. *Part B:* For each set, compute the deviations from the set means (x_s). For example, the first score in set 1 of part A is 146; the deviation of this score from the mean of set 1 is: $146 - 140.7 = 5.3$. Actually, it is not necessary to record the signs, as shown, as these values will be squared.

TABLE 1-1
One-way Analysis of Variance Problem:
Body Weights of Advanced, Normal, and Retarded
Maturity Groups

A. *Body Weights* (*pounds*)

	Set 1 Advanced	Set 2 Normal	Set 3 Retarded
	146	117	76
	128	96	61
	127	101	59
	150	109	78
	141	99	91
	180	108	87
	116	99	80
	140	92	81
	141	79	74
	138	83	82
ΣX_s	1407	983	769
M_s	140.7	98.3	76.9

$$\Sigma X_t = 3159$$
$$M_t = 105.3$$

B. *Deviations Within Sets* (x_s)

+ 5.3	+18.7	− 0.9
−12.7	− 2.3	−15.9
−13.7	+ 2.7	−17.9
+ 9.3	+10.7	+ 1.1
+ 0.3	+ 0.7	+14.1
+39.3	+ 9.7	+10.1
−24.7	+ 0.7	+ 3.1
− 0.7	− 6.3	+ 4.1
+ 0.3	−19.3	− 2.9
− 2.7	−15.3	+ 5.1

C. *Squares of Deviations Within Sets* (x^2)

28.09	349.69	0.81
161.29	5.29	252.81
187.69	7.29	320.41
86.49	114.49	1.21
0.09	0.49	198.81
1544.49	94.09	102.01
610.09	0.49	9.61
0.49	39.69	16.81
0.09	372.49	8.41
7.29	234.09	26.01

$$\Sigma x_s^2 = 4781.10 \qquad (SS)_w$$

D. *Deviations of Set Means from Total Mean* (*d*)

d	35.4	−7.0	−28.4
d^2	1253.16	49.0	806.56
nd^2	12531.6	490.0	8065.6

$$\Sigma d^2 = 2108.72$$
$$n\Sigma d^2 = 21087.2 \qquad (SS)_b$$

However, a check can be made on the accuracy of this step by adding each column; all sums should be zero.

3. *Part C:* Square the deviations within sets. For example, the first entry in set 1 of part B is 5.3; this amount squared equals 28.09. Add all squares; in this problem, Σx_s^2 is 4781.10. This amount is the *SS* for within sets.

4. *Part D:* For the *d* row, compute d_s for each set: $M_s - M_t$. The mean of set 1 in part A is 140.7; the total mean is 105.3. Thus, for this set: $d = 140.7 - 105.3 = 35.4$. As a check, the sum of this row should equal zero, as all deviations are taken from the M_t of 105.3. In the second row, these values are squared (d^2); the sum of the row is 2,108.72. By multiplying this amount by n: $n\Sigma d^2 = 10 \times 2,108.72 = 21,087.2$. The third row merely checks this out by multiplying each d^2 by 10 and adding. This amount is the *SS* for between sets.

5. The next step is to obtain the mean squares for the within-sets and between-sets variances; the formulas followed are 1.2 and 1.3 respectively. The following tabulations will facilitate this process:

Variances	SS	df	MS
Within sets	4781.10	27	177.08
Between sets	21087.20	2	10,543.60

Thus, $(MS)_w = 177.08$; and $(MS)_b = 10,543.60$.

6. The *F* ratio is now computed as the ratio between the two mean squares. The between sets mean square becomes the numerator for this ratio:

$$F = \frac{(MS)_b}{(MS)_w} = \frac{10,543.60}{177.08} = 59.54$$

7. The *F* ratio of 59.54 for this problem is unusually large; without a doubt, it is highly significant. In order to determine significance, however, consult Table A in the Appendix. Enter the column of this table with *df* of the between-sets mean square. Since there are 2 degrees of freedom for this variance, select column 2. Enter the row with *df* of the within-sets mean square—in this case 27. Where column 2 and row 27 meet, the required *F*s for significance at the .05 and .01 levels are 3.35 and 5.49. The obtained *F* of 59.54 is much greater than 5.49; therefore, the null hypothesis is rejected well beyond the .01 level.

SET MEANS OF UNEQUAL SIZE

In the problem above, set means are of equal size, with 10 subjects each. Usually studies utilizing analysis of variance in the treatment of data are planned so the set means are of equal size; the computation is simpler and, as will be seen later, more post hoc methods of testing the significance of differences between paired means following a significant F ratio are available. However, circumstances may prevent such an equalization of the number of subjects in the sets. When such occurs, the procedure of computing $n\Sigma d^2$ in Table 1-1, part D, last line, is followed, since it allows for differences in set n's.

SIGNIFICANCE OF DIFFERENCE BETWEEN PAIRED MEANS

As indicated earlier, the F ratio tests the significance of the differences between the means of several samples. If the F test is insignificant, the solution of the problem is completed. The null hypothesis is automatically accepted for the differences between all sets of paired means; thus, the differences found between the means can be attributed to sampling error. If the F ratio is significant, the null hypothesis is automatically rejected for the greatest difference between any pair of means, regardless of what subsequent tests of significance may show. If the F ratio just reaches significance at the level accepted, this one difference will probably be the only significant one. However, if the F ratio is appreciably larger than the level accepted, other differences between pairs of means may also be significant. Quite frequently, the investigator will want to know if other differences between pairs of means are significant and for which differences the null hypothesis may be rejected.

Early in the use of analysis of variance, the t test was used to evaluate the difference between each pair of set means when the F ratio was significant. The primary limitation in following this practice is that it increases the probability of a Type I error, i.e., rejecting the null hypothesis when in fact it is true. Lindquist[3] has explained this situation by stating:

> In applying a simple t test to a difference between the means of two independent samples, we read from the table of t the probability that the observed value of t would be exceeded in any single randomly selected instance if the null hypothesis were true. The probability that a single randomly selected difference will exceed a given value, however, is by no means the same as the probability that the *largest of a number* of randomly selected differences will exceed this value.

In analysis of variance with several randomly established groups, this latter situation prevails. For additional comments on this situation refer to the beginning of this chapter.

Therefore, the probability of rejecting the null hypothesis when it is actually true increases with the number of intergroup means being tested for

[3] E. T. Lindquist, *Design and Analysis of Experiments in Psychology and Education* (Boston: Houghton-Mifflin Company, 1953), pp. 48–49.

significance. When the number of comparisons is large, the number of decisions that potentially can be wrong because of Type I error can be relatively large. Nelson and Morehouse[4] summarize the seriousness of this situation by stating that the probability of committing a Type I error "increases from .05 for two groups to .13 when all possible comparisons are made for three groups, .22 with four groups, and .40 with five an so on." Thus, multiple t tests are inappropriate for the purpose of testing the significance of differences between the means of paired sets following a significant analysis of variance F ratio.

After the overall F ratio has been found significant, then a comparison between any pair of means may be made. In this case, unlike that of planned comparison between two means (t ratio), the requirement that such *post hoc* comparisons must be independent is not in effect. Usually, the investigator will be interested in examining all pairs of means, but any comparison is legitimate.

Inasmuch as the t ratio is inappropriate in making tests of significance when more than two means are involved, a number of proposals have been advanced for making such comparisons. Winer[5] contrasted the power of the following five methods for making post hoc tests of significance between paired means: Duncan multiple range test, Newman-Keuls test, Tukey's extension of Fisher's least significant difference (LSD) procedure, Tukey's honestly significant difference (HSD) method, and the Scheffé S test. He concluded that the Scheffé test has the greatest power and is most conservative with respect to Type I error; this method leads to the smallest number of significant differences. The Tukey HSD method is also a stringent test of significance, with the LSD being slightly less stringent. The Duncan multiple range test and the Newman-Keuls method are the least powerful tests. The applications of four of these methods will be given below: Scheffé, Tukey HSD, Newman-Keuls, and Duncan tests.

SCHEFFÉ S TEST[6]

The Scheffé S method has a number of advantages for testing the significance of post hoc differences between means, as follows: applicable to groups of unequal sizes; suitable for any comparison between means or the comparison of the average of two or more means with other means; linked closely with the F test and requires only the F table in performing computations; robust under non-normality and heterogeneous variance conditions;

[4] Richard C. Nelson and Chauncey A. Morehouse, "Statistical Procedures Used in Multiple-Group Experiments," *Research Quarterly 37*, no. 3 (October 1966): 441.

[5] B. J. Winer, *Statistical Principals in Experimental Design* (New York: McGraw-Hill Book Company, 1962), p. 88.

[6] H. A. Scheffé, "A Method of Judging All Possible Contrasts in the Analysis of Variance," *Biometrika 4* (1953): 87–104.

strong test of significance. The basic procedure in the Scheffé method is to compute the limits of a confidence interval for each difference between means.

In the one-way analysis problem presented in Table 1-1, the F ratio was 59.54; the three weight means of the advanced, normal, and retarded maturity groups were 140.7, 98.3, and 76.9 pounds respectively. The process of testing the significance of the differences between all pairs of means by the Scheffé method follows. Some adaptations for simplicity are made, but these adaptations in no way change the computations or, thus, the answer obtained.

1. The formula for computing the amount of the confidence interval (I) is:

$$I = S\sqrt{(MS)_w Wg} \qquad (1.4)$$

2. Compute: $\sqrt{(MS)_w Wg}$ in which

$(MS)_w = MS$ within-sets variance

$\qquad\quad = 177.08$ (computed in analysis of variance problem)

and $\qquad Wg = \dfrac{1}{n} + \dfrac{1}{n}$ (function of n of sets)

$$\qquad\qquad = \dfrac{1}{10} + \dfrac{1}{10} = \dfrac{1}{5}$$

therefore $\sqrt{(MS)_w Wg} = \sqrt{177.08/5} = 5.95$

3. Compute $S = \sqrt{(k-1)(F_{.05})}$ or $\sqrt{(k-1)(F_{.01})}$ (function of confidence levels) in which $k =$ number of columns and $F_{.05}$ and $F_{.01}$ are F ratios needed for significance at the .05 and .01 levels obtained from Table A.

Therefore, at the .05 level:

$$S = \sqrt{(k-1)(F_{.05})} = \sqrt{(3-1)(3.35)} = 2.59$$

and at the .01 level:

$$S = \sqrt{(k-1)(F_{.01})} = \sqrt{(3-1)(5.49)} = 3.31$$

4. Complete formula 1.4:

.05 level: $S\sqrt{(MS)_w Wg} = (2.59)(5.95) = 15.41$

.01 level: $\qquad\qquad\qquad = (3.31)(5.95) = 19.69$

5. If a difference between means equals or exceeds the confidence interval for a given level, the difference is significant. The weight means in order of magnitude and the differences between these means for the maturity groups in the foregoing analysis of variance problem are given in Table 1-2.

All differences between means are significant inasmuch as they exceed the I of 19.69.

TABLE 1-2
*Ordered Weight Means and Differences between Means
for Maturity Groups in One-way Analysis of Variance Problem*

Means (in pounds)			Differences
Advanced	*Normal*	*Retarded*	*between Means*
140.7	98.3		42.4
140.7		76.9	63.8
	98.3	76.9	21.4

TUKEY HSD METHOD[7]

In using Tukey's honestly significant difference (HSD) method for post hoc testing of the differences between paired means following a significant analysis of variance F ratio, the n's of the sets must be equal or approximately so. The difference between two means is significant if it exceeds HSD. The formula for computing HSD is:

$$HSD = q\sqrt{\frac{(MS)_w}{n}} \qquad (1.5)$$

in which $(MS)_w$ is the mean square for within-sets variance in the analysis of variance problem; n is the set mean. The value of q is obtained from the distribution of the studentized range statistic, as given in Table B in the appendix. The sampling distribution of q is based on the fact that the range of random samples becomes larger as the sample size increases. In order to enter Table B, two values are needed: df for $(MS)_w$ and k.

The computational procedures for the Tukey HSD method will be illustrated from the foregoing analysis of variance problem. In this problem: $(MS)_w = 177.08$; $n = 10$. To obtain q from Table B, enter column 3, which is k for this problem, and row 27, which is the df for $(MS)_w$. The q's at the .05 and .01 levels are 3.51 and 4.50, respectively. Thus, at the .01 level, using formula 1.5:

$$HSD = 4.50\sqrt{\frac{177.08}{10}}$$

$$= 4.50 \times 4.21$$

$$= 18.95$$

[7] J. W. Tukey, *The Problem of Multiple Comparisons* (Mimeograph, Princeton University, 1953). Also, see Roger E. Kirk, *Experimental Design: Procedures for the Behavioral Sciences* (Belmont, Calif.: Brooks/Cole Publishing Company, 1969), p. 88.

All differences between means in the problem as shown in Table 1-2, are larger than 18.95, so these differences are significant at the .01 level and beyond.

NEWMAN-KEULS TEST[8]

The Newman-Keuls test for determining the significance of the differences between paired means is a modified q statistic. The critical amounts for significance changes for this method, depending upon the number of ordered means between the pairs of means being compared. The general formula is:

$$W_r = q_r\sqrt{\frac{(MS)_w}{n}} \qquad (1.6)$$

where q_r is obtained from the distribution of studentized range statistic (Table B in the appendix). The subscript r designates the number of steps separating means arranged in order of magnitude: for adjacent means, the r is 2; for each intervening mean, the r increases by 1.

For the ordered weight means in this problem, as shown in Table 1-2, $r = 2$ for the adjacent means of the advanced and normal and the normal and retarded maturity groups. For the q_r for these comparisons, enter column 2 and row 27, the df for $(MS)_w$, of Table B; the amount at the .01 level is 3.93. Applying formula 1.6:

$$W_2 = 3.93\sqrt{\frac{177.08}{10}} = 16.55$$

The difference between the adjacent means are 42.4 and 21.4 pounds, so these differences are significant above the .01 level.

For the comparison of the means of the advanced and retarded groups, r is 3, as one mean intervenes in the ordered sequence of means. For the q_r for this comparison, enter column 3 and row 27; the amount at the .01 level is 4.50. Applying formula 1.6:

$$W_3 = 4.50\sqrt{\frac{177.08}{10}} = 18.95$$

The difference between the means of these groups is 63.8 pounds, so significance is obtained well beyond the .01 level.

---

[8] M. Keuls, "The Use of Studentized Range in Connection with Analysis of Variance," *Emphytica* (1952).

DUNCAN MULTIPLE RANGE TEST[9]

The Duncan multiple range test is similar to the Newman-Keuls method for testing the significance of the differences between paired means. The only computational difference between the methods is in the table used to obtain the q values.

For adjacent means in the ordered sequence of means, the q values are the same for both methods. However, when means intervene in the ordered sequence, the "protection level," as Duncan calls it, increases less and the q becomes smaller than for the Newman-Keuls test. Duncan has argued that if k is greater than 2, there is a greater chance for real differences to exist than when k is only equal to 2. In other words, he does not give as much credence to the presence of intervening means in an ordered series as does the Newman-Keuls process.

The same formula (1.6) is used with the Duncan and the Newman-Keuls tests. The q values are obtained from Table C in the appendix. When $r = 2$, the results of these two methods are the same. Thus, the r's are 2.90 and 3.93 at the .05 and .01 levels; and the W_2 at the .01 level is 16.55. For $r = 3$, enter column 3 and row 27; q's are 3.05 and 4.10 at the two levels. To compute W_3 at the .01 level apply formula 1.6:

$$W_3 = q_r\sqrt{\frac{(WS)_w}{n}}$$

$$= 4.10\sqrt{\frac{177.08}{10}} = 17.26$$

The difference between the means of groups C and A, with the intervening mean for group B, is 63.8 pounds, as shown in Table 1-2, which far exceeds the W_3 of 17.26 required for significance at the .01 level.

COMPARISONS

As indicated above, the power of the various methods for testing the significance between paired means following a significant analysis of variance F ratio varies with the method used. This fact may be illustrated with the results obtained from applying the four methods above. The critical values at the .01 level for the three methods are shown in Table 1-3.

As can be seen, the difference between means must be greatest for significance when the Scheffé S test is used. The Tukey HSD and Newman-Keuls methods produce the same critical values when $r = k$. The Duncan multiple range test is the least stringent test of significance: The critical values

[9] D. B. Duncan, "Multiple Range and Multiple F Tests," *Biometrics*, 11, no. 1 (March 1955): 1–42.

TABLE 1-3
Comparison of Post Hoc Tests of Significance
for Differences between Paired Means in Analysis of Variance

| | | k or r |
Methods	2	3
Scheffé S Test	19.69	19.69
Tukey HSD Method	18.95	18.95
Newman-Keuls Test	16.55	18.95
Duncan Multiple Range Test	16.55	17.26

are the same for a given $(df)_w$ by Newman-Keuls and Duncan methods when $r = 2$; these values, however, decrease consistently with the number of intervening means in a numerically ordered sequence.

Two-Way Analysis of Variance

In one-way analysis of variance, only one experimental factor was involved. Thus, in the illustrated problem, the differences in mean weights for three maturity groups were tested for significance. In two-way analysis of variance, two experimental factors are studied. An example previously mentioned is the whirlpool bath study by Badgley, in which the effects of varying the temperature of the water and the length of time the foot was in the water upon the range of motion of the ankle joint were determined. Other examples are the effects of varying weights and cadences upon work done on an elbow flexion ergograph and variations in hand and foot placements upon speed in sprint starting.

To illustrate computation of two-way analysis of variance, the differences between the mean wights of 12-year-old boys grouped by skeletal age and standing height are tested for significance. Three maturity groups compose the columns (k) and three standing height groups compose the rows (r). Thus, nine combinations (sets), known as interaction (i) of maturity and standing height groups are formed; five subjects (n) are included in each set.

Four sources of variance are found in two-way analysis of variance: between columns, between rows, interaction, and residual. The residual variance is the within-sets variance as identified in the preceding one-way classification problem. This variance is the amount remaining after the other three sources of variance have been removed. It is sometimes called the error variance for the reason that it represents the influences of unknown and uncontrolled forces. Three F tests are made for the differences between the means of the columns, of the rows, and of interaction. The residual variance serves as the denominator for all F tests, and so plays a very important part in determining the significance of the variances tested.

A computational model is presented below for calculating the two-way analysis of variance. The following symbols are used:

k: Particular column
r: Particular row
X_{ij}: Any score in row r and column k
M_{rk}: Any set mean
n: Number within each set
x_t: Deviation of any X_{ij} from M_t

PROBLEM COMPUTATION

The data for this problem are contained in Table 1-4. The steps in making the computations follow.

TABLE 1-4
Two-Way Analysis of Variance Problem:
Body Weights of Three Maturity and Three Height Groups

Standing Heights	Advanced	Maturity Groups Normal	Retarded	Sums for Heights	Means for Heights
Tall	125	147	89		
	129	120	80		
	140	128	106		
	139	116	98		
	118	125	109		
Σ	651	636	482	1769	
M	130.2	127.2	96.4		117.93
Average	55	133	137		
	91	120	94		
	121	112	114		
	119	140	109		
	117	102	98		
Σ	547	607	· 552	1706	
M	109.4	121.4	110.4		113.73
Short	117	125	80		
	110	137	100		
	96	132	71		
	72	106	109		
	93	119	62		
Σ	488	619	422	1529	
M	97.6	123.8	84.4		101.93
Σ for Skeletal Age	1686	1862	1456	5004	
M for Skeletal Age	112.40	124.13	97.07		111.20

1. Compute the means of all columns, rows, sets, and the total mean (M_t). These are shown in Table 1-4, in which $M_t = 111.20$ pounds.

2. Compute the total sum of squares from the following formula:

$$\Sigma x_t^2 = \Sigma(X_{ij} - M_t)^2 \tag{1.7}$$

To illustrate with first and last rows in Table 1-4:

First row: $(125 - 111.20)^2 + (147 - 111.20)^2 + (89 - 111.20)^2$

$+ \dots\dots\dots\dots\dots\dots\dots\dots\dots\dots\dots\dots\dots\dots\dots$

Last row: $+ (93 - 111.20)^2 + (119 - 111.20)^2 + (62 - 111.20)^2$

$= (13.8)^2 + (35.8)^2 + (-22.2)^2$

$+ \dots\dots\dots\dots\dots\dots\dots\dots\dots\dots\dots\dots\dots\dots\dots$

$+ (-18.2)^2 + (7.8)^2 + (-49.2)^2$

$= 190.64 + 1{,}281.64 + 492.84$

$+ \dots\dots\dots\dots\dots\dots\dots\dots\dots\dots\dots\dots\dots\dots\dots$

$+ 331.24 + 60.84 + 2{,}420.64$

$= 17{,}697.20$

3. Compute SS between rows from the following formula:

$$\Sigma d_r^2 = nk[\Sigma(M_r - M_t)^2] \tag{1.8}$$

$= (5)(3)[(117.93 - 111.20)^2 + (113.73 - 111.20)^2$

$\qquad + (101.93 - 111.20)^2]$

$= 15[(6.73)^2 + (2.53)^2 + (-9.27)^2]$

$= 15 \times 137.63$

$= 2{,}064.45$

4. Compute SS between columns from the following formula:

$$\Sigma d_k^2 = nr[\Sigma(M_k - M_t)^2] \tag{1.9}$$

$= (5)(3)[(112.40 + 111.20)^2 + (124.13 - 111.20)^2$

$\qquad + (97.06 - 111.20)^2]$

$= 15[(1.20)^2 + (12.93)^2 + (-14.13)^2]$

$= 15 \times 368.28$

$= 5{,}524.20$

5. Compute SS for interaction by a two-step process. The steps and respective formulae are:

a. Compute SS for rows, columns, and interaction from the following formula:

$$\Sigma d_{rk}^2 = n[\Sigma(M_{rk} - M_t)^2] \tag{1.10}$$

$$
\begin{aligned}
&= 5[(130.2 - 111.2)^2 + (127.2 - 111.2)^2 + (96.4 - 111.2)^2 \\
&\quad + (109.4 - 111.2)^2 + (121.4 - 111.2)^2 + (110.4 - 111.2)^2 \\
&\quad + (97.6 - 111.2)^2 + (123.8 - 111.2)^2 + (84.4 - 111.2)^2] \\
&= 10,055.00
\end{aligned}
$$

b. Compute interaction SS using the following formula:

$$
\begin{aligned}
\Sigma d_{r \cdot k}^2 &= \Sigma d_{rk}^2 - \Sigma d_r^2 - \Sigma d_k^2 \\
&= 10,055.00 - 2064.45 - 5524.20 \\
&= 2,466.35
\end{aligned}
$$

6. Compute SS for residual (within sets). This computation can be done with the following formula:

$$\Sigma x_s^2 = \Sigma(X_{ij} - M_{rk})^2 \tag{1.12}$$

However, a simple way to obtain the residual SS is to deduct the SSs for the rows, columns, and interaction from the total SS. Thus:

$$17,697.20 - 10,055.00 = 7,642.20$$

7. Determine degrees of freedom as follows:

		This Problem
Between rows	$r - 1$	$3 - 1 = 2$
Between columns	$k - 1$	$3 - 1 = 2$
Interaction	$(r - 1)(k - 1)$	$2 \times 2 = 4$
Residual	$rk(n - 1)$	$(3)(3)(5 - 1) = 36$
Total	$N - 1$	$45 - 1 = 44$

As can be seen, the sum of degrees of freedom for the rows, columns, interaction, and residual variances equals the total degrees of freedom.

8. Compute mean squares for all variances by dividing their respective sum of squares by degrees of freedom. Thus:

Source of Variance	SS	df	MS
Rows: Standing Height	2,064.45	2	1,032.23
Columns: Skeletal Age	5,524.20	2	2,762.10
Interaction	2,466.35	4	616.59
Residual	7,642.20	36	212.28

9. Compute F ratios by dividing the MSs of the rows, columns, and interaction by the MS for residual variance. Thus:

$$F \text{ for standing height:} \quad \frac{1,032.3}{212.28} = 4.86$$

$$F \text{ for skeletal age:} \quad \frac{2,762.10}{212.28} = 13.01$$

$$F \text{ for interaction:} \quad \frac{616.59}{212.28} = 2.90$$

10. Determine significance of F ratios. Enter Table A. For each F ratio, enter the column with df for the variance being tested and the row with df for the residual variance. In this problem, the row is 36, the residual df, for all F ratios; the columns are 2 for standing height and skeletal age and 4 for interaction. From this table, the F ratios required for significance are:

	Level	
	.05	.01
Standing height	3.26	5.25
Skeletal age	3.26	5.25
Interaction	2.64	3.89

The F ratio of 13.01 obtained for the differences between the mean weights of the skeletal age groups is significant well beyond the .01 level, so the null hypothesis can be rejected with assurance. The differences in mean weights for the standing height groups nearly reached significance at the .01 level, since this F ratio was 4.86. The F ratio for interaction is significant at the .05 level ($F = 2.90$).

POST HOC TESTS OF SIGNIFICANCE

A test to determine the significance between all pairs of means where F ratios are significant is next applied. Some differences exist between applying tests of significance to the rows and columns and applying them to interaction. The process for the columns and rows follows.

Scheffé Test. In this problem, the F ratios for both columns and rows were significant. Inasmuch as k and r are the same—each 3—a single computation will suffice to determine the confidence interval for all tests of significance; where these differ, separate computations are necessary. In each instance, $n = 15$, as each row contains three maturity groups of 5 each and each column contains three height groups of 5 each. Thus, using formula 1.4, as for the one-way analysis of variance:

$$I = S\sqrt{(MS)_w Wg}$$

in which $(MS)_w = 212.28$, the residual MS in the problem, and

$$Wg = \frac{1}{n} + \frac{1}{n}$$

$$= \frac{1}{15} + \frac{1}{15} = \frac{1}{7.5}$$

therefore

$$\sqrt{(MS)_w Wg} = \sqrt{\frac{212.28}{7.5}} = \sqrt{28.30} = 5.32$$

and

$$S = \sqrt{(k-1)(F_{.05})} = \sqrt{(3-1)(3.26)} = 2.55*$$
$$S = \sqrt{(k-1)(F_{.01})} = \sqrt{(3-1)(5.25)} = 3.24*$$

Complete the formula:

.05 level: $S\sqrt{(MS)_w Wg} = (2.55)(5.32) = 13.57$

.01 level: $= (3.24)(5.32) = 17.24$

Thus, the limits of the confidence intervals for the differences between the weight means of columns and rows in this problem are determined from 13.57 and 17.24 at the .05 and .01 levels respectively.

The weight means by order of magnitude and the differences between these means for the maturity and height groups in the two-way analysis of variance problem are given in Table 1-5. Applying the I's of 13.57 and 17.24 to the differences between the means of the maturity groups (Part A) shows that the retarded group has significantly lower means than the normal group at the .01 level and than the advanced group at the .05 level; the difference between the weight means of the normal and the advanced groups is 11.73 pounds, so it was not significant. Making the same application to the height

* *Note:* The S formula for rows is: $\sqrt{(r-1)(F)}$. In this problem r and k are the same, so one computation serves both situations. If r was 4, $r - 1 = 3$. Further, the F from Table A in the Appendix, pp. 122–24, also changes, as $df = 3$, so column 3 is entered.

groups, we see that the weight mean of the tall group is significantly higher—
near the .01 level—than the mean of the short group; therefore, the other
differences between means are not significant.

TABLE 1-5
Ordered Weight Means and Differences Between Means
for Maturity and Height Groups
in Two-Way Analysis of Variance Problem

	Means (in pounds)		Mean Difference
	Part A: Maturity Groups		
Normal	Advanced	Retarded	
124.13	112.40		11.73
124.13		97.06	27.07
	112.40	97.06	15.34
	Part B: Height Groups		
Tall	Normal	Short	
117.93	113.73		4.20
117.93		101.93	16.00
	113.73	101.93	11.80

Tukey HSD Method. For the Tukey HSD method, formula 1.5
is utilized, as follows:

$$\text{HSD} = q\sqrt{\frac{(MS)_w}{n}}$$

As for one-way analysis of variance, the value for q is obtained from Table B
in the appendix. The column of this table is entered with k or r of 3, inasmuch
as the problem contains the same number of rows and columns; the row in
Table B is 36, the df for the residual or within-sets variance. Thus, the
q values at the .05 and .01 levels are 3.46 and 4.40, respectively. Substituting
in the formula:

$$.05 \text{ level:} \quad \text{HSD} = 3.46\sqrt{\frac{212.28}{15}} = 13.01$$

$$.01 \text{ level:} \quad \text{HSD} = 4.40\sqrt{\frac{212.28}{15}} = 16.54$$

By this method, all differences between the weight means for the three
maturity groups are significant or nearly so at the .05 level, as seen from
Table 1-5. The smallest difference between paired means is 11.73 pounds for
the advanced and normal groups; this difference does not reach the HSD of
13.01 needed for significance at this level. The .01 level of significance is

exceeded for the mean difference of 27.07 pounds for the normal and retarded groups.

The weight mean for the short group is significantly lower at the .05 level than the means of the tall and normal groups; the mean differences are 16.00 and 11.80 pounds, respectively. The difference between the means of the tall and normal groups is not significant.

Newman-Keuls Test. Formula 1.6 is utilized for the Newman-Keuls test:

$$W_r = q_r \sqrt{\frac{(MS)_w}{n}}$$

As before, the value for q_r is obtained from Table B in the appendix. Columns 2 and 3 are entered, inasmuch as there are 3 means each for columns and for rows; the row in Table B is 36, the df for residual variance. Thus, the q_r values are 2.87 and 3.46 at the .05 level. Substituting in the formula:

$$W_2 = 2.87 \sqrt{\frac{212.28}{15}} = 10.79$$

$$W_3 = 3.46 \sqrt{\frac{212.28}{15}} = 13.01$$

For the ordered weight means for the maturity groups in this problem, as shown in Table 1-5, Part A, the differences between means of adjacent maturity groups are 11.73 pounds for normal and advanced groups and 15.34 pounds for advanced and retarded groups; these amounts exceed the W_2 of 10.79, and so are significant at the .05 level. The difference between the weight means of the normal and retarded groups, where a mean intervenes, is 27.07 pounds; this amount exceeds considerably the W_3 of 13.01, so is significant well beyond the .05 level (and the .01 level although not shown here). For the ordered height groups (Part B), the differences between adjacent weight means are 4.20 pounds for tall and normal groups and 11.80 pounds for normal and short groups; only the difference between the latter two groups reached the W_2 needed for significance at the .05 level. The difference of 16.00 pounds between the tall group and the short group exceeded the W_3 of 13.01, and so is also significant at the .05 level.

Duncan Multiple Range Test. For the Duncan multiple range test, formula 1.6 is used, as for the Newman-Keuls test above. However, the q is obtained from Table C; this table is entered in the same way as Table B. Thus, columns 2 and 3 are entered, inasmuch as there are three means each for columns and for rows; the row is 36, the df for residual variance. Thus, the q_r values are 2.86 and 3.00 at the .05 level for r's 2 and 3, respectively.

W_2 will not be calculated, as it is the same amount (10.79) as for the Newman-Keuls test. However:

$$W_3 = 3.02\sqrt{\frac{212.28}{15}} = 11.38$$

Applying the W_2 of 10.79 and the W_3 to the differences between the ordered means in Table 1-5, the same differences between means are significant at the .05 level as for the Newman-Keuls test.

INTERACTION

Computation. Interaction variations are those attributed to the two main effects factors acting together rather than to the main effects factors acting separately. Therefore, in order to obtain the true interaction between the experimental factors in a two-way analysis of variance, variations attributed to the two factors separately are removed. In Table 1-4 some set means are much higher than others. For example, the weight means for the advanced maturity-tall height set and for the retarded maturity-short height set are 130.2 and 84.4 pounds respectively; the difference is 45.8 pounds. However, this difference may be due to the effects of the separate factors, advanced-retarded maturity and tall-short heights.

To remove these separate effects, the matrix of set means is manipulated so that all rows and columns equal the total mean. The matrix of set means, taken from Table 1-4, is given in Table 1-6. The total mean is 111.2 pounds; two steps are necessary to bring the weight means of all rows and columns to this amount.

1. *Columns:* Obtain the difference between each column mean in Part A and the total mean; add this difference to each set mean in the column. The mean of the first column is 112.4; the difference between this mean and the total mean is $111.2 - 112.4 = -1.2$. Subtract this amount from each set mean in the column and enter the amount in Part B. For example, for the first set mean: $130.2 - 1.2 = 129.0$. When this operation is completed, the mean of the column equals the total mean.

Continue in the same manner for the other two columns, first calculating the amount each column mean deviates from the total mean. These amounts are:

Normal column: $111.2 - 124.1 = -12.9$ (subtract from
                                                                                each set mean)

Retarded column: $111.2 - 97.1 = 14.1$ (add to each set mean)

In Part B, all column means equal the total mean of 111.2. The row means, however, have not changed.

TABLE 1-6

Interaction Variance in Two-Way Analysis Variance:
Removal of Separate Weight Variances Contributed Separately
by Maturity and Height

Row (Height)	Advanced	Normal	Retarded	Σ	M
	Columns (Skeletal Age)				
		A. Original Matrix of Set Means			
Tall	130.2	127.2	96.4	353.8	117.9
Average	109.4	121.4	110.4	341.2	113.7
Short	97.6	123.8	84.4	305.8	101.9
Σ	337.2	372.4	291.2	1,000.8	
M	112.4	124.1	97.1		111.2
		B. Removal of Variations Associated with Skeletal Age			
Tall	129.0	114.3	110.5	353.8	117.9
Average	108.2	108.5	124.5	341.2	113.7
Short	96.4	110.9	98.5	305.8	101.9
Σ	333.6	333.7	333.5	1,000.8	
M	111.2	111.2	111.2		111.2
		C. Removal of Variations Associated with Height			
Tall	122.3	107.6	103.8	333.7	111.2
Average	105.7	106.0	122.0	333.7	111.2
Short	105.7	120.2	107.8	333.7	111.2
Σ	333.7	333.8	333.6	1,001.1	
M	111.2	111.2	111.2		111.2

2. *Rows:* Obtain the difference between each row mean and the total mean; add this difference to each set mean in the row (Part B). The mean of the first row is 117.9; the difference between this mean and the total mean is $111.2 - 117.9 = -6.7$. Subtract this amount from each set mean in the row and amount in Part C. For example, for the first row mean: $129.0 - 6.7 = 122.3$. When this operation is completed, the mean of the row equals the total mean.

Continue in the same manner for the other two rows, first calculating the amount by which each row mean deviates from the total mean. These amounts are:

Average row: $111.2 - 113.7 = -2.5$ (subtract from each set mean)

Short row: $111.2 - 101.9 = 9.3$ (add to each set mean)

In Part C, all row means now equal the total mean. In fact, all row and column means are the same as the total mean.

The F ratio for interaction analysis was 2.90, which is just significant

at the .05 level. If this ratio had not been significant, the above manipulation
of the matrix of means would not have been done, since the null hypothesis
could have been accepted for all interaction differences between means. With
a minimal F ratio (2.90), the largest difference between interaction-manipula-
ted means (Table 1-6, Part C) is significant at the .05 level. This largest
difference is 18.47 pounds, between the advanced-tall set (122.27 pounds) and
the retarded-tall set (103.80 pounds). Post hoc comparisons between pairs of
set means would be pointless in this situation.

Interaction Illustration. Guilford[10] provides a clearer illustration of
the effects of separate experimental factors in an interaction situation. In
this experiment, the subjects threw at targets of four sizes by use of three machines. Thus, the two experimental factors were target size and machine used,
a two-way classification problem in which 12 sets were evident. The original
matrix of means resulting from this experiment appears in Table 1-7, Part A.

TABLE 1-7
*Interaction of Means
for Various Targets and Machines*

Row	Machines 1	2	3	Σ	M
	*A. Original Matrix of Means*				
A	4	3	2	9	3
B	5	5	2	12	4
C	7	6	5	18	6
D	8	6	7	21	7
Σ	24	20	16	60	
M	6	5	4		5
	*B. Means after Removal of Separate Variances*				
A	5	5	5	15	5
B	5	6	4	15	5
C	5	5	5	15	5
D	5	4	6	15	5
Σ	20	20	20	60	
M	5	5	5		5

In examining the matrix of original means (Table 1-4, Part A), higher
means obviously occur as the target size is increased from A to D. Some sets
had means three to four times higher than the means in other sets. Yet the
interaction F ratio was insignificant: .97, when 2.30 was needed for signifi-

[10] J. P. Guilford, *Fundamental Statistics in Psychology and Education*, 4th ed.
(New York: McGraw-Hill Book Company, 1965), p. 295.

cance at the .05 level. The respective F ratios for the targets and machines were 15.00 and 5.85, both significant at and beyond the .01 level.

The variances associated with the targets and machines separately were removed by the procedure described above; the resulting matrix of means is shown in Table 1-4, Part B. Obviously, little interaction exists and this is insignificant as was already known from the F ratio of .97. The size of the target was the dominant factor in this experiment, although some variance related to the machines was also evident; these two factors, however, did not function in combination.

Comments on Analysis of Variance

As explained, analysis of variance is used to test the null hypothesis that no true differences exist among a number of means. Or, stated differently, the F ratio tests the hypothesis that all groups compared are actually random samples from the same normally distributed population. If the F ratio is not significant, the null hypothesis is accepted; if the F ratio is significant, the differences between means are larger than those which might occur from sampling errors; the samples do not come from the same population.

Typically, a number of assumptions have been advocated when analysis of variance is used to test the significance of the differences between several means. These assumptions are:

1. The sampling within sets is random.
2. The variances within sets are approximately equal.
3. Observations within sets are from normally distributed populations.
4. The contributions to total variance are additive.

However, extensive studies by Norton[11] on sampling distributions as related to analysis of variance have cast considerable doubt on the rigidity with which these assumptions must be met. With artificial populations of 10,000, he varied the shapes of distributions in several ways, including normal leptokurtic, rectangular, markedly skewed, and J-shaped. Further, he changed the variances of normal populations from 25 to 100 to 225; the standard deviations were 5, 10, and 15, respectively.

Norton concluded that the F ratio is rather insensitive to differences in the shape of population distributions. This observation is consistent with the principle that distributions of sample means approach normality even though the populations from which they are drawn are not normally distributed. Further, Norton found that the F ratio was somewhat insensitive to differences in population variances, and that only marked differences are serious.

[11] Reported in E. F. Lindquist, *Design and Analysis of Experiments in Psychology and Education* (Boston: Houghton Mifflin Company, 1953), pp. 78–90.

Extension of Analysis of Variance

Analysis of variance can be used much more extensively than is presented in this book, in which one-way and two-way analyses are described. These analyses can be extended to higher order classifications, such as the three-way and four-way. Using the whirlpool bath study by Badgley[12] mentioned earlier in this chapter, the various orders up to three will be illustrated.

One-way analysis of variance could be computed by studying the effect of one experimental factor at a time. Thus, the effect of varying water temperature on ankle joint range of motion could have been determined by keeping the time the foot was in the water constant for all treatments. Similarly, the effects of various times could be evaluated by keeping the water temperature constant for all treatments.

Badgley, however, chose to vary systematically both factors—water temperature and time foot was immersed—in combination; consequently, his data were treated as a two-way analysis of variance. If he had added a third factor in combination with the others, such as the force with which the water circulated, he would have appropriately performed a three-way analysis of variance.[13]

Additional Illustrated Problems

Although illustrations of studies in which analysis of variance has been used in the analysis of data are evident in the problems used in the computational examples above, additional descriptions of research of this nature will be presented in the following paragraphs.

ONE-WAY ANALYSIS OF VARIANCE

Academic Achievement of Athletes. In the Medford, Oregon, Boys' Growth Project, Stafford[14] compared the academic achievement of elementary and junior high school athletes and nonparticipants; both single-year and longitudinal analysis were made. Academic achievement was evaluated by standard achievement tests and grade point average. At the close of each sport's season, the coaches rated the athletic ability of each member of their squads in football, basketball, baseball, track, and wrestling. The

---

[12] Badgley, "A Study of the Effect of the Whirlpool Bath."

[13] For example of three-way analysis of variance problem, see Quinn McNemar, *Psychological Statistics*, 3rd ed. (New York: John Wiley and Sons, Inc., 1962), pp. 318–38. McNemar also presents other uses of analysis of variance.

[14] Elba G. Stafford, "Single-Year and Longitudinal Comparisons of Intelligence and Academic Achievement of Elementary and Junior High School Athletes and Nonparticipants," Microcard Doctoral Dissertation, University of Oregon, 1968.

following rating scale, as abbreviated, was used: *3*, outstanding athlete; *2*, regular player; *1*, substitute; *NP*, nonparticipant.

The statistical application for this study was one-way analysis of variance whereby the differences between the academic achievement means of the various athletic and nonparticipant groups were tested for significance. In those instances where a significant *F* test provided evidence of overall significance among means, the Scheffé *S* method to test for significant differences between paired means was used.

For 12-year-old athletes, the most consistently significant *F* ratios were obtained for Language Usage on the Stanford Achievement Test. These *F* ratios were collected from the thesis for the various interscholastic sports as shown in Table 1-8. All *F* ratios are significant beyond the .05 level, as they exceed the 2.43 to 2.67 ratios needed for significance at this level.

TABLE 1-8

Analysis of Variance for Language Usage of 12-year-old Nonparticipants and Athletes in Various Sports

| *Sports* | *NP* | *Means* | | | | *Mean Squares* | | |
		1	*2*	*3*	*Within*	*Between*	*F Ratio*
Football	7.45	8.54	7.99	12.63	27.93	92.45	3.42
Basketball	7.45	6.88	8.14	16.50	26.04	142.86	5.49
Baseball	7.45	8.55	7.07	14.74	26.89	114.05	4.24
Track	7.45	7.85	7.90	13.86	27.47	94.48	3.44

Upon application of the Scheffé *S* test to the differences between paired means, the confidence intervals for the various *df* ranged from 1.91 to 3.24 at the .05 level. Only the 3-rated athletes in all sports were found to have significantly higher means in Language Usage than the other rated athletes and nonparticipants. This situation is illustrated in Table 1-9 for the football players.

TABLE 1-9

Scheffé Test for Language Usage Variances for 12-year-old Nonparticipants and Football Players

| *Means* | | | | |
3	*2*	*1*	*NP*	*Difference in Means*
12.63	7.98			4.65*
12.63		8.54		4.09*
12.63			7.44	5.19*
	7.98	8.54		−.56
	7.98		7.44	.54
		8.54	7.44	1.10

* *Significant at .05 level and beyond.*

Other Studies. In addition to the examples of research in which one-way analysis of variance was employed in the anlysis of data, other illustrations are briefly offered to provide the student with wider acquaintance of its applicability.

Carron[15] studied the effects of fatigue on the ability to learn a motor skill. Seventy-five college women were assigned to three equal groups and given 25 trials on a pursuit rotor. One group was given a fatiguing arm task early in learning (trial 6), a second group was fatigued late in learning (trial 15), and a third group served as a control, receiving no interpolated fatigue. All subjects received 25 additional trials without the application of fatigue on a second day. A one-way analysis of variance applied to the differences between the means on initial performances was not significant, since the F ratio was only .68. When the effects of fatigue upon performance were examined, F ratios of 3.37 and 14.38 were obtained between means of the three groups when the interpolation of physical fatigue early and late respectively in the practice session. Application of the Duncan multiple range test on the paired means indicated in both early and late fatigue situations that the group receiving fatigue had significantly poorer motor performances.

To assess the effect of training on cardiovascular adjustment to gravity, Shvartz[16] assigned 33 male subjects to three equal groups. One of these groups was trained for seven weeks by means of pull-ups and dips; a second group trained through bench stepping; the third group served as a control. Orthostatic tolerance before and after training was determined by heart rate and blood pressure differences between horizontal and standing and between horizontal and vertical positions on a tilt board. These data were analyzed by analysis of either variance or covariance. The decision of which analysis to use in the various situations was made as follows: Pretraining measures were plotted against post-training measures for the three groups; if the regression lines of the three groups were essentially parallel, analysis of variance was used; if the plotted lines were not parallel, analysis of covariance was applied. The significant results were: (1) The trained individuals had a smaller increase in heart rate and a smaller decrease in pulse pressure than did the control group. (2) Comparison between the two trained groups revealed that the group which trained using upper body exercise had a smaller decrease in pulse pressure upon tilting.

TWO-WAY ANALYSIS OF VARIANCE

Whirlpool Bath Study. Inasmuch as reference has been made repeatedly to the "whirlpool bath" study by Badgeley,[17] additional details pertaining

[15] Albert V. Carron, "Physical Fatigue and Motor Learning," *Research Quarterly* 40, no. 4 (December 1969): 682.

[16] Esar Shavartz, "Effect of Two Different Training Programs on Cardiovascular Adjustments to Gravity," *Research Quarterly 40*, no. 3 (October 1969): 575.

[17] Badgley, "A Study of the Effect of the Whirlpool Bath."

to this study will be given to illustrate a two-way analysis of variance problem. The purpose of the study was to determine the effects of different water temperatures and immersion times upon the flexion-extension range of motion of the ankle joint. The temperatures were 82, 92, 102, and 112 degrees; the times were 4, 12, 20, and 28 minutes. The number of subjects was 7 for each of the 16 situation, a total of 112. The ankle flexion-extension movement of each subject was measured with a goniometer before and after his whirl-pool bath. The difference between the post- and pre-means for the 7 subjects in each experimental situation constituted the result of the bath on ankle flexibility. The matrix of mean differences is shown in Table 1-10.

TABLE 1-10
Mean Differences in Ankle Flexibility
Before and After Whirlpool Baths

Bath Times	*Water Temperatures*				
	82°	*92°*	*112°*	*128°*	*Total*
4 Minutes	−4.57	−4.14	2.00	3.71	−0.75
12 Minutes	−1.57	−5.14	6.00	5.00	1.07
20 Minutes	−1.43	−2.43	−0.57	3.29	−0.29
28 Minutes	−2.73	−2.57	−2.00	2.14	−1.29
Total	−2.58	−3.57	1.36	3.54	−0.31

The F ratios resulting from the anlysis of variance were: 30.62 for temperatures, significant well beyond the .01 level; 2.85 for times, significant at the .05 level; 1.78 for interaction, insignificant at the .05 level. Since this study was done a number of years ago, the t ratio was used to test the significance between paired means. All differences between means for the temperatures were significant at and beyond the .01 level, except for the difference between 82° and 92°. Only one time difference between means—the difference between 12 and 28 minutes—was significant at the .05 level.

Thus, ankle flexibility became greater as a result of whirlpool baths when the temperature of the water increased from 92° to 112°. As a general observation, too, water temperature below body temperature restricted range of motion, whereas the reverse was noted for water temperature over body temperature. Time in the water from 4 to 28 minutes had little effect on ankle range of motion. The interaction was insignificant; thus the combinations of temperature and time did not prove effective under the conditions of the experiment.

Other Studies. An example of a two-way analysis of variance is provided in a portion of a study by Drowatzky,[18] whose primary aim was to

[18] John N. Drowatzky, "Effects of Massed and Distributed Practice Schedules upon the Acquisition of Pursuit Rotor Tracking by Normal and Mentally Retarded Subjects," *Research Quarterly 41*, no. 1 (March 1970): 32.

compare the effects of massed versus distributed practice on the rate of build-up or dissipation of reactive inhibition affecting the acquisition of a motor skill. The experiment was designed in such a way that reminiscence could also be examined. Thirty normal and 29 mentally retarded subjects were randomly assigned to three groups, each of which received 400 seconds for one of the following pursuit rotor practice schedules: massed practice, 20-second intertrial rest, and 2-minute intertrial rest. After the first series of trials the subjects had 5 minutes of rest, and then received further trials. Analysis of variance revealed significant differences between the tracking ability of normal and retarded subjects, between massed and distributed practice, between trials, and for several combinations of interaction effects. A two-way analysis of variance was computed for reminiscence (defined as the difference between the last prerest and the first postrest score); no significant difference existed between normal and retarded subjects, but massed versus distributed practice and the interaction between the two sets of variables were significantly different. The findings suggested that trainable mentally retarded individuals may be penalized by being given massed practice during the early stages of learning.

In one phase of his experiment, Straub[19] studied the effect of using warm-up throwing drills employing a systematic overload procedure on speed and accuracy of the overarm baseball throw. Sixty subjects were placed into high velocity and low velocity groups and further divided into three subgroups of 10 subjects each. These three subgroups were given maximal preliminary throwing trials utilizing either regulation size, 10-ounce, or 15-ounce weighted baseballs. They were then tested for the immediate effects of overload warm-up on throwing velocity by means of a two-way analysis of variance. The only significant F ratio was a high 49.20 for the differences between postoverload velocity level means. This result was attributed to the "built in" or matching aspect of the study. Thus, the overload treatments were ineffective in producing significant increments in throwing velocity: Control subjects who warmed up exclusively with regulation baseballs threw just as fast as those subjects who received 10-ounce or 15-ounce weighted ball warm-ups.

[19] William F. Straub, "Effect of Overload Training Procedures upon Velocity and Accuracy of the Overarm Throw," *Research Quarterly 39*, no. 2 (May 1968): 370.

2

ANALYSIS
OF
COVARIANCE

In the conduct of studies in which experimental factors are applied, experimental and control groups can be formed in various ways. In setting up an experiment, the investigator may form a control and one or more experimental groups by equating or matching. In both instances, the initial means and standard deviations are essentially alike. The formation of equated groups requires a person-to-person matching of subjects based on scores made on the essential test used for this purpose. For matched groups, person-to-person equating is not done, but the subjects are so arranged that the means and standard deviations of the groups are comparable.

Equivalent groups, whether formed by equating or matching, are not always easy to develop. The formation of such groups usually necessitates a reduction in the size of N in order to obtain reasonably close matches. To put it another way, a larger number of subjects must be tested on the matching variable in order to secure groups of adequate size when matching is performed. Furthermore, in the matched-group method, it is often difficult to obtain the correlation between the matching and experimental variables for the population from which the samples are drawn.

$$\sigma_{DM} = \sqrt{(\sigma_{M_1}^2 + \sigma_{M_2}^2)(1 - r_{xy}^2)}$$

For a random-group experiment, the means of the groups will be different, except by merest chance, as a consequence of drawing random samples from the same population. Sampling theory and sampling process are discussed in chapter 10 of *Research Processes*.[1] From a review of this material, it will be obvious that the means of repeated independent samples of the same size drawn by chance from the same population will differ from each other in accordance with the laws of normal probability.

[1] David H. Clarke and H. Harrison Clarke, *Research Processes in Physical Education, Recreation, and Health* (Englewood Cliffs, N.J.: Prentice-Hall, Inc., 1970).

The fact, then, that initial (pre-experiment) means will differ from each other, even though the difference is not significant—and therefore can be attributed to sampling error—may well affect the significance of the differences between final (post-experiment) means. For example:

	Group A	Group B	Difference
Initial means	32	35	3
Final means	41	38	3
Mean gains	9	3	6

Assuming that the difference of 3 each between the initial means and between the final means is not significant, the investigator could erroneously conclude that the difference between the effects of his experiment are unimportant. However, on the average, Group A gained 9 points whereas Group B increased only 3 points, a mean difference of 6 points. Quite probably, the difference between mean gains is significant, since Group A made three times the increase of Group B.

One way to treat these experimental data is to test the difference in mean gains for significance. A generally more acceptable way, however, is to apply analysis of covariance. In analysis of covariance, the final means are adjusted for differences in initial means, and the adjusted means are tested for significance. A further advantage of this method is that analysis of variance is first computed for the differences between initial means. In this instance, a non-significant F ratio will provide confidence that the initial samples came from the same population—and are devoid of sampling bias.

Analysis of Covariance Problem

COMPUTATION

Analysis of covariance may be computed for any number of experimental groups. In the analysis to follow, a control and two experimental groups were utilized. As one phase of a study by Macintosh,[2] the effects of isometric and isotonic exercises on the development of elbow flexion strength was investigated. Three groups of 20 college men each were formed by random selection. The control group did not exercise the elbow flexors during the experimental period of eight weeks; one experimental group engaged in isometric exercises and the other experimental group participated in isotonic exercises

[2] Donald D. Macintosh, "The Relationship of Individual Differences and Subsequent Changes in Static Strength with Speed of Forearm Flexion Movement," (Microcard doctoral dissertation, University of Oregon, 1964).

of these muscles. The strength of the muscles was tested by tensiometer methods at the start and end of the experiment. The data were treated by analysis of covariance, for which the process is described below.[3]

1. *Prepare Table 2-1.* In the table X_1, X_2, and X_3 are the initial scores of the subjects; Y_1, Y_2, and Y_3 are their corresponding final scores. The cross products (XY) of the scores are computed and entered in the third column of each section, designated A, B, and C for each of the three groups: control, isometric, and isotonic, respectively. Each of the columns is added and the means of the X's and Y's are computed. At the bottom of the table, the results of the following additional computations are given for the *three groups combined*: ΣX, ΣY, ΣX^2, ΣY^2, and ΣXY.

TABLE 2-1

Illustrated Problem: Analysis of Covariance for Control and Experimental Isometric and Isotonic Groups (Strength Tested in Kilograms)

Group A: Control			Group B: Isometric			Group C: Isotonic		
X_1	Y_1	$X_1 Y_1$	X_2	Y_2	$X_2 Y_2$	X_3	Y_3	$X_3 Y_3$
80	86	6880	71	86	6106	72	86	6192
66	58	3828	78	83	6474	76	77	5852
73	77	5621	57	64	3648	57	77	4389
69	69	4761	57	69	3933	74	89	6586
59	60	3540	48	48	2304	59	67	3953
73	68	4964	62	60	3720	73	88	6424
62	70	4340	60	66	3960	56	62	3472
63	58	3654	59	60	3540	54	63	3402
73	74	5402	71	83	5893	56	68	3808
55	60	3300	66	64	4224	66	77	5082
68	69	4692	53	58	3074	80	83	6640
66	72	4752	71	80	5680	65	80	5200
66	67	4422	47	50	2350	58	70	4060
56	57	3192	73	80	5840	55	61	3355
65	69	4485	80	95	7600	51	60	3060
62	69	4278	61	82	5002	63	67	4221
83	83	6889	64	70	4480	65	73	4745
66	64	4224	62	67	4154	56	72	4032
60	69	4140	71	77	5467	71	83	5893
62	69	4278	64	67	4288	63	80	5040
Σ 1327	1368	91642	1275	1409	91737	1270	1483	95406
M 66.4	68.4		63.7	70.5		63.5	74.2	

For All 3 Groups:

$\Sigma X = 3872$ $\Sigma Y = 4260$

$\Sigma X^2 = 253882$ $\Sigma Y^2 = 308508$ $\Sigma XY = 278785$

---

[3] This computation pattern follows the one described in the following reference: Henry E. Garrett, *Statistics in Psychology and Education*, 6th ed. (New York: Donald McKay Company, Inc., 1966), pp. 295–303. (As will be noted, analysis of variance is computed in a different manner from the one described in Chapter 1.)

2. *Correction terms* (c). Prepare three correction terms for X, Y, and XY of the three groups combined. The formulas and computations follow.

$$c_x = \frac{(\Sigma X)^2}{N} = \frac{(3872)^2}{60} = 249873$$

$$c_y = \frac{(\Sigma Y)^2}{N} = \frac{(4260)^2}{60} = 302460$$

$$c_{xy} = \frac{(\Sigma X)(\Sigma Y)}{N} = \frac{(3872)(4260)}{60} = 274912$$

In which, $N = 60$, the total N for the problem.

3. *Total SS*. The total SS for X, Y, and XY for all groups combined are computed. The formula and computations are:

$$SS_x = \Sigma X^2 - c_x = 253882 - 249873 = 4009$$

$$SS_y = \Sigma Y^2 - c_y = 308508 - 302460 = 6048$$

$$SS_{xy} = \Sigma XY - c_{xy} = 278785 - 274912 = 3873$$

4. *Between group means SS*. The between group SS for x, y, and xy are computed from the following formulas:

$$x = \frac{X_1^2 + X_2^2 + X_3^2}{n} - c_x = \frac{1327^2 + 1275^2 + 1270^2}{20} - 249873 = 100$$

$$y = \frac{Y_1^2 + Y_2^2 + Y_3^2}{n} - c_y = \frac{1368^2 + 1409^2 + 1483^2}{20} - 302460 = 340$$

$$xy = \frac{(X_1 Y_1) + (X_2 Y_2) + (X_3 Y_3)}{n} - c_{xy}$$

$$= \frac{(1327)(1368) + (1275)(1409) + (1270)(1483)}{20} - 274912 = -151$$

5. *Within groups SS*. The within groups SS for x, y, and xy are found by subtracting the among means SS from the SS_t. Thus:

$$x = 4009 - 100 = 3909$$

$$y = 6048 - 340 = 5708$$

$$xy = 3873 - (-151) = 4024$$

6. *Analysis of variance*. An analysis of variance of the X and Y scores taken separately is next computed. The following computations show this process from the calculations so far completed:

Source of Variance	df	SS_x	SS_y	$MS_x(V_x)$*	$MS_y(V_y)$†
Between Means $(k - 1)$	2	100	340	50.0	170.0
Within Groups $(N = k)$	57	3909	5708	68.6	100.1
Total	59	4009	6048		

* *Divide SS_x by df.*

$$F_x = \frac{50.0}{68.6} = 0.73$$

† *Divide SS_y by df.*

$$F_y = \frac{170.0}{100.1} = 1.70$$

Consulting Table A in the appendix with df's of 2 and 57, the F ratios needed for significant differences between the means are 3.16 and 5.08 at the .05 and .01 levels, respectively. The F test applied to the initial scores ($F_x = 0.73$) falls short of significance at the .05 level, so it is demonstrated that the X means do not differ significantly and that the random assignment of subjects to the two groups was successful. The F ratio for the final (Y) means was not significant either, since the F ratio of 1.70 did not reach the 3.70 needed for significance at the .05 level. However, this lack of significance could be due to the differences in initial means. Therefore, the covariance process continues.

7. *Compute adjusted SS.* This step leads to the computation of covariance and the F ratio for the differences among the final adjusted means, through computation of adjusted SS for Y. The symbol $SS_{y \cdot x}$ indicates that SS_y has been adjusted for any variability in Y contributed by X; in other words, SS of the final scores are adjusted for differences in SS of the initial scores. The general formula is:

$$SS_{y \cdot x} = SS_y - \frac{(SS_{xy})^2}{SS_x}$$

In which S_{xy} is the SS_{xy} for the adjusted total and within groups SS, respectively. Thus:

$$\text{Total } SS = SS_y - \frac{(SS_{xy})^2}{SS_x} = 6048 - \frac{(3873)^2}{4009} = 2306$$

$$\text{Within } SS = SS_y - \frac{(SS_{xy})^2}{SS_x} = 5708 - \frac{(4024)^2}{3909} = 1566$$

The between groups SS is obtained by subtraction.

$$\text{Between } SS = 2306 - 1566 = 740.$$

8. *Computation of covariance.* The analysis of covariance is computed in the same manner as analysis of variance, except the adjusted SS are used. Thus:

Source of Variance	df	SS_x	SS_y	S_{xy}	$SS_{y \cdot x}$	$MS_{y \cdot x}$*	$SD_{y \cdot x}$†
Between Sets	2	100	340	−151	740	370	
Within Sets	56‡	3909	5708	4024	1566	28	5.29
Total	58	4009	6048	3873	2306		

* *Divide $SS_{y \cdot x}$ by df.*
† $SD_{y \cdot x} = \sqrt{(MS_{y \cdot x})w} = \sqrt{28} = 5.29$
‡ *1 more df lost in covariance analysis: $N - k - 1$.*

The F ratio is computed from the adjusted MS's:

$$F = \frac{(MS_{y \cdot x})_b}{(MS_{y \cdot x})w} = \frac{370}{28} = 13.2$$

Enter Table A with 2 and 56 *df* to determine the F ratios required for significance; these ratios are 3.16 and 5.01 at the .05 and .01 levels, respectively. Thus, the differences among the three final adjusted means are significant well beyond the .01 level, since the F ratio obtained is 13.2. The value of covariance becomes apparent from this problem. The final means before adjustment for differences in initial means did not vary significantly from each other, as indicated by the analysis of variance F ratio of 1.70; when the final means were adjusted, the F ratio was definitely significant.

The final adjustment means have not been determined, as the analysis of covariance was calculated from the adjusted sum of squares. If the F ratio is not significant, nothing would be gained by computing the adjusted means. Since the F ratio is significant, the process should continue.

9. *Correlation.* The correlations between the x and y values (the initial and final scores) may be computed from the adjusted amounts in step 8; however, the r's are not needed in future computations. The process will be explained in case such correlations are wanted for other purposes, and for the additional understanding they provide. The following general formula is applied to the appropriate SS's for total, between means, and within groups:

$$r = \frac{\Sigma xy}{\sqrt{\Sigma x^2 \cdot \Sigma y^2}} = \frac{S_{xy}}{\sqrt{(SS_x)(SS_y)}}$$

Thus, from the amounts in the table given in step 8:

$$\text{Total } r = \frac{3873}{\sqrt{(4009)(6048)}} = 0.79$$

$$\text{Between Means } r = \frac{-151}{\sqrt{(100)(340)}} = -0.82$$

$$\text{Within } r = \frac{4024}{\sqrt{(3909)(5708)}} = 0.85$$

The within-groups correlation of .85 shows a better relationship between initial and final scores than does the total correlation of .79, although the difference is not great. In this situation, systematic differences in means have been eliminated from the within r. The high correlation between X and Y accounts for the marked significance between Y means when adjusted for variability in X. A high correlation within groups reduces the denominator of the variance ratio ($F_{y \cdot x}$); a low correlation between X and Y means would proportionately affect the numerator.

10. *Regression score weights.* Regression coefficients (b) for total, among means, and within groups are next computed.[4] The general formula is:

$$b = \frac{\Sigma xy}{\Sigma x^2} = \frac{S_{xy}}{SS_x}$$

Thus, from the amounts in the table appearing in step 8:

$$\text{Total } b = \frac{3873}{4009} = 0.97$$

$$\text{Between Means } b = \frac{-151}{100} = -1.51$$

$$\text{Within } b = \frac{4024}{3909} = 1.03$$

The within b is the most nearly unbiased estimate of the regression of X on Y, since any systematic influence due to differences between means has been removed. Therefore, this regression weighting is used in the computation of the adjusted Y means in the following step.

11. *Adjusted Y Means.* The following tabulation shows the initial, final, and adjusted final kilogram means for the three groups in this problem.

[4] Regression coefficients are considered in chapter 4.

Groups	n	M_x	M_y	$M_{y \cdot x}$
A. Control	20	66.4	68.4	66.4
B. Isometric	20	63.7	70.5	71.3
C. Isotonic	20	63.5	74.2	75.2
General Means	60	64.5	71.0	71.0

The adjusted means are computed from the following formula:

$$M_{y \cdot x} = M_y - b_w(M_x - \text{Gen. } M_x)$$

Thus, for the three groups:

Group A $M_{y \cdot x} = 68.4 - 1.03(66.4 - 64.5) = 66.4$

Group B $M_{y \cdot x} = 70.5 - 1.03(63.7 - 64.5) = 71.3$

Group C $M_{y \cdot x} = 74.2 - 1.03(63.5 - 64.5) = 75.2$

SIGNIFICANCE BETWEEN PAIRED ADJUSTED FINAL MEANS

The same post hoc methods of testing the significance of the differences between paired means following a significant analysis of variance F ratio can be applied to the differences between paired adjusted final means after a significant covariance F ratio. Adjustments need only be made to the equivalent covariance values, as indicated in the computations by use of a prime symbol. The adjusted strength means in order of magnitude and the differences between these means for the control and two experimental groups in the above analysis of covariance problem are given in Table 2-2.

TABLE 2-2
Ordered Adjusted Strength Means and Differences
between Means for Control and Experimental Groups
in Analysis of Covariance Problem

Means (kilograms)			
C Group	B Group	A Group	Mean Differences
75.2	71.3		3.9
75.2		66.4	8.8
	71.3	66.4	4.9

In this problem: $n = 20$; $k = 3$; $(df)'_w = N - k - 1 = 60 - 3 - 1 = 56$. In making the computations, the adjusted within-sets mean square $(MS)'_w$ is also needed. Inasmuch as $(SS)'_w$ is 1566 (step 7) and $(df)'_w$ is 56:

$$(MS)'_w = \frac{1566}{56} = 28.00$$

Scheffé S Test. The Scheffé S test described in chapter 1 in the analysis of variance problem (formula 1.4) may be used for testing the significance between paired adjusted means. However, the Scheffé method can also be expressed as an F ratio, as will be shown here. The general formula for these computations is:

$$F' = \frac{(M'_1 - M'_2)^2}{(MS)'_w\left(\frac{1}{n} + \frac{1}{n}\right)} \qquad (2.1)$$

Applying the formula to the paired adjusted means:

$$F'_{M_c - M_a} = \frac{(M'_c - M'_a)^2}{(MS)'_w\left(\frac{1}{n} + \frac{1}{n}\right)} = \frac{(75.2 - 66.4)^2}{28\left(\frac{1}{20} + \frac{1}{20}\right)} = \frac{77.44}{2.8} = 27.66$$

$$F'_{M_b - M_a} = \frac{(M'_b - M'_a)^2}{(MS)'_w\left(\frac{1}{n} + \frac{1}{n}\right)} = \frac{(71.3 - 66.4)^2}{28\left(\frac{1}{20} + \frac{1}{20}\right)} = \frac{24.01}{2.8} = 8.58$$

$$F'_{M_c - M_b} = \frac{(M'_c - M'_b)^2}{(MS)'_w\left(\frac{1}{n} + \frac{1}{n}\right)} = \frac{(75.2 - 71.3)^2}{28\left(\frac{1}{20} + \frac{1}{20}\right)} = \frac{15.21}{2.8} = 5.43$$

In order to be significant, F' must equal $(k - 1)(F_{.05}$ or $F_{.01})$, indicated in step 8, the F ratios from Table A in the appendix for this problem are 3.16 and 5.01 at the .05 and .01 levels. Thus, the necessary F' ratios for the differences between paired adjusted means, inasmuch as $k - 1$ is $3 - 1$, or 2, are:

.05 level: $2 \times 3.16 = 6.32$

.01 level: $2 \times 5.10 = 10.02$

Referring to the tabulation of differences between adjusted strength means in Table 2-2, group A has a significantly lower mean than the means of groups C at the .01 level and B at the .05 level. The difference between the means of groups B and C is not significant.

Tukey HSD Method. The formula for Tukey's honestly significant difference (HSD) method applied to the difference between paired adjusted means is:

$$HSD = q\sqrt{\frac{(MS)'_w}{n}} \qquad (2.2)$$

The value of q is obtained from the distribution of the studentized range statistic, as given in Table B in the appendix. Enter the column for k and the row for $(df)'_w$; these amounts are 3 and 56 in this problem. From the table, the q's are 3.41 and 4.34 at the .05 and .01 levels. Applying the formula:

$$.05 \text{ level:} \quad \text{HSD} = 3.41\sqrt{\frac{28}{20}} = 4.03$$

$$.01 \text{ level:} \quad \text{HSD} = 4.34\sqrt{\frac{28}{20}} = 5.12$$

Referring to the tabulation of differences between adjusted strength means in Table 2-2, the Tukey HSD method also revealed that the mean of group A was significantly lower than the means of groups C and B at the .01 and .05 levels respectively, and that the difference between the means of groups B and C was not significant.

Newman-Keuls Test.   The Newman-Keuls formula applied to the differences between paired adjusted means following a significant covariance F ratio is:

$$W_r = q_r\sqrt{\frac{(MS)'_w}{n}} \tag{2.3}$$

The subscript r designates the ordered positions of the magnitude of the adjusted means. For adjacent means, the r is 2; when one mean intervenes, the r is 3. Enter Table B in the appendix to obtain the q values: the column for r and the row for $(df)'_w$; for this problem, columns 2 and 3 and row 56. The computations follow.

For r = 2:

$$.05 \text{ level:} \quad W_2 = 2.83\sqrt{\frac{28.0}{20}} = 3.34$$

$$.01 \text{ level:} \quad W_2 = 3.75\sqrt{\frac{28.0}{20}} = 4.43$$

For r = 3:   When $r = k$, as in this problem, the results of the Newman-Keuls test are the same as for the Tukey HSD method. Thus: $W_3 =$ 4.03 and 5.10 at the .05 and .01 levels.

In the tabulation of ordered adjusted strength means given in Table 2-2, the means of groups C and B and groups B and C are adjacent; the group C mean is significantly higher than the group B mean at the .05 level and the group B mean is significantly higher than the group A mean at the .01 level. The W_2 values needed at these levels are 3.34 and 4.43; the differences between the adjusted means were 3.9 and 4.9 kgms., respectively. The mean for group C was significantly higher than the group A mean well beyond the .01 level; the required W_3 is 5.10, while the difference between the adjusted means was 8.8 kgms.

Duncan Multiple Range Test. The formula for the Duncan multiple range test applied to the differences between paired adjusted means is the same as for the Newman-Keuls test. The only computational difference between the methods is in the use of Table C in the Duncan procedure. The computations are:

For r = 2: When $r = 2$, the results of the Newman-Keuls and the Duncan tests are the same. Thus: $W_2 = 3.35$ and 4.43 at the .05 and .01 levels, respectively.

For r = 3:

$$.05 \text{ level: } \quad W_3 = 2.98\sqrt{\frac{28.0}{20}} = 3.50$$

$$.01 \text{ level: } \quad W_3 = 3.93\sqrt{\frac{28.0}{20}} = 4.64$$

For the tabulation in Table 2-2, the pattern of significant differences between adjusted strength means is the same as for the Newman-Keuls test.

Control of Covariates

In the first part of this chapter, an important application of analysis of covariance for experimental research, whether used in physical education, another field of education, or psychology, was made. As indicated, it is especially appropriate and convenient when the equation of the control and experimental groups either cannot be accomplished or it is difficult or impractical to do so for various reasons. Although not as frequently found in phsycial education research, control of one or more covariate—or con-comitant—factors can also be achieved through analysis of covariance. In this situation, the assumption is that the covariate and experimental (criter-ion) factors are well related, i.e., have a significant degree of covariance.

COMPUTATION

The following hypothetical example will explain the meaning of this application of analysis of covariance and will illustrate the computational procedures. Three randomly formed groups of eight subjects each were taught handball by three different methods. The subjects were beginners in the sport, so a pre-test of handball ability was not administered. Before the subjects were instructed under their respective methods, however, they were given a motor educability test. These data were used to adjust handball achievement scores obtained at the conclusion of the experiment for differences in the motor educability of the subjects. The process of computing analysis of covariance under these circumstances follows; the data are fictitious with scores kept small for ease of illustration.

Step 1: Prepare Table 2-3. In the table, X_1, X_2, and X_3 are the motor educability scores obtained by the subjects prior to the experiment; Y_1, Y_2, and Y_3 are their corresponding handball scores at the end of the experiment. The X and Y columns for each of the three groups are squared, as shown respectively in adjacent columns. The cross products of the scores (XY's) are computed and appear in the last column under each method. Each of the columns is added; the sums are shown in the row designated by the symbol, Σ. At the bottom of the table, the results of the following additional computations appear for the three groups combined: $\Sigma X, \Sigma Y, \Sigma X^2, \Sigma Y^2,$ and ΣXY.

TABLE 2-3
Illustrated Problem: Analysis of Covariance
Showing Control of Concomitant Factor

		Method 1					Method 2					Method 3		
X_1	X_1^2	Y_1	Y_1^2	$X_1 Y_1$	X_2	X_2^2	Y_2	Y_2^2	$X_2 Y_2$	X_3	X_3^2	Y_3	Y_3^2	$X_3 Y_3$
4	16	7	49	28	4	16	8	64	32	3	9	6	36	18
2	4	5	25	10	5	25	9	81	45	2	4	9	81	18
4	16	6	36	24	5	25	7	49	35	2	4	7	49	14
2	4	4	16	8	4	16	8	64	32	3	9	8	64	24
3	9	5	25	15	3	9	7	49	21	4	16	8	64	32
2	4	4	16	8	1	1	5	25	5	4	16	7	49	28
5	25	7	49	35	2	4	6	36	12	2	4	6	36	12
6	36	8	64	48	5	25	8	64	40	6	36	9	81	54
Σ 28	114	46	280	176	29	121	58	432	222	26	98	60	460	200

For All Three Groups:

$\Sigma Xs = 83$ $\Sigma X^2s = 333$ $\Sigma Ys = 164$ $\Sigma Y^2s = 1172$ $\Sigma XYs = 598$

Step 2: Within-Sets Error Terms. Within-sets error terms are computed below; the data are taken from Table 2-3.

Method 1

$\Sigma xx_1 = \Sigma X_1^2 - [(\Sigma X_1)^2/n] = 114 - [(28)^2/8] = 16.00$

$\Sigma yy_1 = \Sigma Y_1^2 - [(\Sigma Y_1)^2/n] = 280 - [(46)^2/8] = 15.50$

$\Sigma xy_1 = \Sigma XY_1 - [(\Sigma X_1)(\Sigma Y_1)/n] = 176 - [(28)(46)/8] = 15.00$

Method 2

$$\Sigma xx_2 = \Sigma X_2^2 - [(\Sigma X_2)^2/n] = 121 - [(29)^2/8] = 15.87$$
$$\Sigma yy_2 = \Sigma Y_2^2 - [(\Sigma Y_2)^2/n] = 432 - [(58)^2/8] = 11.50$$
$$\Sigma xy_2 = \Sigma XY_2 - [(\Sigma X_2)(\Sigma Y_2)/n] = 222 - [(29)(58)/8] = 11.75$$

Method 3

$$\Sigma xx_3 = \Sigma X_3^2 - [(\Sigma X_3)^2/n] = 98 - [(26)^2/8] = 13.50$$
$$\Sigma yy_3 = \Sigma Y_3^2 - [(\Sigma Y_3)^2/n] = 460 - [(60)^2/8] = 10.00$$
$$\Sigma xy_3 = \Sigma XY_3 - [(\Sigma X_3)(\Sigma Y_3)/n] = 200 - [(26)(60)/8] = 5.00$$

Total

$$\Sigma xx_t = \Sigma xx_1 + \Sigma xx_2 + \Sigma xx_3 = 16.00 + 15.87 + 13.50 = 45.37$$
$$\Sigma yy_t = \Sigma yy_1 + \Sigma yy_2 + \Sigma yy_3 = 15.50 + 11.50 + 10.00 = 37.00$$
$$\Sigma xy_t = \Sigma xy_1 + \Sigma xy_2 + \Sigma xy_3 = 15.00 + 11.75 + 5.00 = 31.75$$

Step 3: Total Variance. Total variances are next obtained, utilizing data found in Table 2-3.

For x

$$1x = \Sigma X_s^2/N = 83^2/24 = 287.04$$
$$2x = \Sigma X_s^2 = 333$$
$$3x = (\Sigma X_1^2 + \Sigma X_2^2 + \Sigma X_3^2)/n = (28^2 + 29^2 + 26^2)/8 = 287.63$$

For y

$$1y = \Sigma Y_s^2/N = 164^2/24 = 1120.65$$
$$2y = \Sigma Y_s^2 = 1172$$
$$3y = (\Sigma Y_1^2 + \Sigma Y_2^2 + \Sigma Y_3^2)/n = (46^2 + 58^2 + 60^2)/8 = 1135.00$$

For xy

$$1xy = [(\Sigma X_s)(\Sigma Y_s)]/N = [(83)(164)]/24 = 567.17$$
$$2xy = \Sigma XY_s = 598$$
$$3xy = [(\Sigma X_1)(\Sigma Y_1) + (\Sigma X_2)(\Sigma Y_2) + (\Sigma X_3)(\Sigma Y_3)]/n$$
$$= [(28)(46) + (29)(58) + (26)(60)]/8 = 566.25$$

Step 4: Sums of Squares. The usual sums of squares needed in analysis of variance and analysis of covariance are computed; these SS are for between (B), within (W), and total (T) variances. The necessary data are taken from Step 3. The $(SS)_t$ in each instance $(Txx, Tyy,$ and $Txy)$ should equal the sum of $(SS)_B$ and $(SS)_W$.

For X

$$Bxx = 3x - 1x = 287.63 - 287.04 = \quad .59$$
$$Wxx = 2x - 3x = 333.00 - 287.63 = 45.37$$
$$Txx = 2x - 1x = 333.00 - 287.04 = \overline{45.96}$$

For Y

$$Byy = 3y - 1y = 1135 - 1120.65 = 14.35$$
$$Wyy = 2y - 3y = 1172 - 1135 \quad\;\; = 37.00$$
$$Tyy = 2y - 1y = 1172 - 1120.65 = \overline{51.35}$$

For XY

$$Bxy = 3xy - 1xy = 566.25 - 567.17 = -.92$$
$$Wxy = 2xy - 3xy = 598 - 566.25 \quad\; = 31.75$$
$$Txy = 2xy - 1yy = 598 - 567.17 \quad\; = \overline{30.83}$$

Step 5: Analysis of Variance.   An analysis of variance can be computed for the differences between mean handball test scores at the end of the experiment. The computation of this F ratio follows, utilizing the Y-data Step 4. The df's are the same as for analysis of variance: $k - 1$ for between sets and $N - k$ for within sets.

Source of Variance	SS	df	MS	F
Between Sets (Byy)	14.35	2	7.18	
Within Sets (Wyy)	37.00	21	1.76	4.08
Total (Tyy)	51.35	23		

For the df's of this problem, enter column 2 and row 21 in Table A of the appendix; the F ratios needed for significance at the .05 and .01 levels are 3.47 and 5.78. Thus, the F ratio of 4.08 is significant at the .05 but not at the .01 level.

Step 6: Analysis of Covariance.   Although the F ratio here indicates significant differences among the means of the methods groups, these differences could conceivably be due to the initial differences between the groups in motor educability. Or, the differences among the means might be greater if differences in motor educability had been controlled at the beginning of the study. Analysis of covariance can compensate statistically for this situation by approximating the results that would have been achieved if the subjects for the three methods groups had been equated on the basis of the concomitant variable. The steps necessary to compute analysis of covariance follow.

In making this computation, the sums of squares are adjusted first for the differences in motor educability scores as follows, utilizing data in Step 4.

$$T'yy = Tyy - [(Txy)^2/Txx] = 51.35 - [(30.83)^2/45.96] = 30.65$$
$$W'yy = Wyy - [(Wxy)^2/Wxx] = 37.00 - (31.75)^2/45.37] = 14.78$$
$$B'yy = T'yy - W'yy = 30.65 - 14.78 = 15.87$$

With these data, the analysis of covariance can be computed, as shown in the following tabulation:

Source of Variance	SS	df	MS	F
Between Sets (B'yy)	15.87	2	7.94	
Within Sets (W'yy)	14.78	20	0.74	10.73
Total (T'yy)	30.65			

The df for between sets remain the same as for analysis of variance in Step 5. However, an additional df is lost in covariance for within sets ($N - k - 1$) so the df in the above computation are 20, instead of 21 as for variance analysis. Thus, entering column 2 and row 20 in Table A in the appendix, the F ratios needed for significance are 3.49 at the .05 level and 5.85 at the .01 level. The significance of the difference between means has increased considerably, from 4.08 in the variance problem to 10.77 in the covariance application.

Step 7: Adjusted Final Means. The final adjusted means, M'_{x_1}, M'_{x_2}, and M'_{x_3}, are computed as follows:

a. Obtain b adjustment coefficient with data from Step 2:

$$b = \Sigma xy_t/\Sigma xx_t = 31.75/45.37 = .70$$

b. From Table 2-3, calculate the means of X and Y for each method and the total mean; enter these means in the first row. Perform the other calculations indicated.

	Set Means (M_s)			Total Mean (M_t)
	Method 1	Method 2	Method 3	
X Means	3.50	3.63	3.25	3.46
$M_s - M_t$	0.04	0.17	−0.21	
Y Means	5.75	7.13	7.50	6.83

The adjusted means (M'_y) are obtained utilizing the following formula:

$$M'_y = M_y - b(M_s - M_t)$$

Applying the formula to the set (methods) means:

Method 1: $M'_{y_1} = 5.75 - (.70)(.04) = 5.72$

Method 2: $M'_{y_2} = 7.13 - (.70)(.17) = 7.01$

Method 3: $M'_{y_3} = 7.50 - (.70)(-.21) = 7.65$

SIGNIFICANCE BETWEEN PAIRED ADJUSTED FINAL MEANS

The same post hoc tests of significance between paired adjusted final means described in the earlier analysis of covariance problem are applied here. In this problem: $n = 8$; $k = 3$; $(df)'_w = 20$; $(MS)'_w = 0.74$. The ordered adjusted handball test means and the differences between these means are given in Table 2-4.

TABLE 2-4
Ordered Adjusted Handball Test Means and Differences between Means
for Three Teaching Methods in Analysis of Covariance Problem

Adjusted Handball Test Means			
Method 3	*Method 2*	*Method 1*	*Mean Differences*
7.65	7.01		.64
7.65		5.72	1.93
	7.01	5.72	1.29

Scheffé F Test. In applying the Scheffé S ratio to determine the significance of paired adjusted handball test means, formula 2.1 is applied, as a general formula:

$$F'_{M_1 - M_2} = \frac{(M'_1 - M'_2)^2}{(MS)'_w \left(\frac{1}{n} + \frac{1}{n} \right)}$$

Applying this formula to the paired adjusted means in Table 2-4:

$$F'_{M_3 - M_1} = \frac{(M'_{y_3} - M'_{y_1})^2}{(MS)'_w \left(\frac{1}{n} + \frac{1}{n} \right)} = \frac{(7.65 - 5.72)^2}{.74 \left(\frac{1}{8} + \frac{1}{8} \right)} = \frac{3.72}{.19} = 20.63$$

$$F'_{M_2 - M_1} = \frac{(M'_{y_2} - M'_{y_1})^2}{(MS)'_w \left(\frac{1}{n} + \frac{1}{n} \right)} = \frac{(7.02 - 5.72)^2}{.74 \left(\frac{1}{8} + \frac{1}{8} \right)} = \frac{1.66}{.19} = 8.74$$

$$F'_{M_3-M_2} = \frac{(M'_{y_3} - M'_{y_2})^2}{(MS)'_w\left(\frac{1}{n} + \frac{1}{n}\right)} = \frac{(7.65 - 7.02)^2}{.74\left(\frac{1}{8} + \frac{1}{8}\right)} = \frac{.40}{.19} = 2.22$$

The F ratios needed for significance is determined by: $(k - 1)(F_{.05}$ or $F_{.01})$. As indicated in Step 6, these F ratios are 3.49 and 5.85 at the .05 and .01 levels. Thus, the necessary F ratios for the differences between paired adjusted means are:

.05 level: $2 \times 3.49 = 7.58$

.01 level: $2 \times 5.85 = 11.70$

In the problem, the adjusted mean for method 1 is significantly lower than the adjusted means of method 3 beyond the .01 level and of method 2 at the .05 level. The difference between the adjusted means for methods 2 and 3 is not significant.

Tukey HSD Method. The formula for the Tukey HSD method of testing significance of the differences between paired adjusted means is the same as before (formula 2.2), as follows:

$$HSD = q\sqrt{\frac{(MS)'_w}{n}}$$

Entering Table B in the appendix with k of 3 and $(df)'_w$ of 20, the q values are 3.58 and 4.64 at the .05 and .01 levels. Applying the formula:

.05 level: $HSD = 3.58\sqrt{\frac{.74}{8}} = 1.11$

.01 level: $HSD = 4.64\sqrt{\frac{.74}{8}} = 1.44$

Referring to the tabulation of differences between adjusted handball test means in Table 2-4, the Tukey and the Scheffé tests agree in designating that the mean of method 1 was significantly lower than the means of methods 3 and 2 at the .01 and .05 levels, respectively, and that the difference between the means of methods 2 and 3 was not significant.

Newman-Keuls Method. The Newman-Keuls formula for testing the differences between paired adjusted means is the same as previously used (formula 2.3), as follows:

$$W_r = q_r\sqrt{\frac{(MS)'_w}{n}}$$

The columns of Table B in the appendix are entered with r's of 2 and 3; the row entry is 20, as before. The computations are:

For r of 2:

$$.05 \text{ level}: \quad W_2 = 2.95\sqrt{\frac{.74}{8}} = .91$$

$$.01 \text{ level}: \quad W_3 = 4.02\sqrt{\frac{.74}{8}} = 1.25$$

For r of 3:   When $r = k$, as in this problem, the results of the Newman-Keuls and the Tukey HSD methods are the same. Thus, $W_3 = 1.11$ and 1.44 at the .05 and .01 levels.

Referring to the tabulation of differences between adjusted handball test means in Table 2-4, the mean of method 1 is significantly lower than the means of both methods 2 and 3 at the .01 level, a change from the results of the Scheffé and Tukey methods. As for the other tests, the difference between the adjusted means of methods 2 and 3 is not significant.

Duncan Multiple Range Test.   The formula for the Duncan multiple range test for determining the significance of differences between paired adjusted means is the same as for the Newman-Keuls test; Table C in the appendix is entered with the same columns and row, as well. The computations are:

For r of 2:   When $r = 2$, the results of the Duncan and Newman-Keuls methods are the same. Thus, $W_2 = .91$ and 1.25 at the .05 and .01 levels.

For r of 3:

$$.05 \text{ level}: \quad W_3 = 3.10\sqrt{\frac{.74}{8}} = .96$$

$$.01 \text{ level}: \quad W_3 = 4.22\sqrt{\frac{.74}{8}} = 1.31$$

Upon referring to Table 2-4, significant differences between paired adjusted handball test means are the same as for the Newman-Keuls test.

Additional Illustrated Problems

An example of the use of the analysis of covariance is provided in a study by Bangerter,[5] who investigated the contribution to the vertical jump made by three groups of leg muscles, the ankle plantar flexors, the knee extensors, and the hip extensors. One hundred subjects were randomly assigned evenly to four experimental groups and a control group. The experimental groups were given progressive resistance training three times per week for eight weeks. Each of three groups excercised one of the three muscle groups; a fourth group performed all of the exercises of the first three groups; the control group did no training. Strength tests and the vertical jumping were administered both before and after the training period. By use of analysis of covariance, the final means of the five groups were adjusted for differences in beginning means; the F ratio for the differences between these adjusted means was 5.39, which exceeded the F of 3.52 needed for significance at the .01 level. The Tukey test was applied to locate the significant differences between paired adjusted final means. Differences were significant between those groups assigned exercises which strengthened the knee and hip extensor muscles, but not for the plantar flexion group or the control group. It is possible that the plantar flexor muscles act not by direct contribution to the vertical jump as do the other muscles, but as stabilizers and resistors to forces that are placed upon them during active jumping.

Hakes and Rosemier[6] studied the relative effectiveness of three time allotments for circuit training and active games in a college physical education program. Three groups were formed as follows: 24 subjects exposed to 5 min. of circuit training and 25 min. of active games; 25 subjects undertook 10 min. of circuit training and 20 min. of active games; 21 subjects, 15 min. of each type of activity. Initial and final tests given to all subjects involved performance on a series of six exercises. An analysis of covariance of final test performance revealed significant differences for three of the exercises (bench steps, leg exchanges, and sit-ups). The Scheffé test showed that the 15-minute allotment to circuit training was better for sit-ups and leg-exchanges than the 5-minute allotment, but the group receiving 10 minutes was significantly superior to the 15-minute group on bench stepping.

[5] Blauer L. Bangerter, "Contributive Components in the Vertical Jump," *Research Quarterly 39*, no. 3 (October 1968): 432.
[6] Richard R. Hakes and Robert A. Rosemier, "Circuit Training Time Allotments in a Typical Physical Education Class Period," *Research Quarterly 38*, no. 4 (December 1967): 576.

Berger and Hardage[7] investigated the question of whether weight training with maximum loads for each of 10 repetitions was more effective for increasing strength than the use of the traditional 10-repetition-maximum (10-RM) procedures. Two groups were employed, both training three times per week for eight weeks on the bench press exercise. Bench press strength (1-RM) was obtained before and after the training period. Analysis of covariance showed that the strength of the two groups was significantly different with the maximum load group having the higher mean. Thus, weight training employing maximum loads for each repetition was more effective for increasing strength than the 10-RM method. Inasmuch as only two groups were employed in the experiment, the F ratio was adequate as the test of significance between final adjusted means; consequently, an application of one of the post hoc tests was not necessary.

[7] Richard A. Berger and Billy Hardage, "Effect of Maximum Loads for Each of Ten Repetitions on Strength Improvement," *Research Quarterly 38*, no. 4 (December 1967): 715.

3

PARTIAL CORRELATION AND MULTIPLE CORRELATION

In considering correlation in the *Research Processes* book only two variables were involved. An extension of correlation to more than two variables will now be considered. In doing so, a simple way of designating the number of variables involved is by *orders*. The former two-variable correlation will be known as zero-order. For each additional variable in the correlation, the order will be increased accordingly. Thus, a first-order correlation would have three variables; a second-order correlation, four variables; and so on. The following advanced methods involving multiple variables in correlation will be presented in this chapter: partial correlation, partial standard deviation, and multiple correlation.

Partial Correlation

MEANING

In determining the correlation between two variables, the investigator may wish to eliminate the influence of other factors which, because of their common relationship to the variables being correlated, obscure or distort correlational results. By means of partial correlation, one or more additional factors may be held constant (partialled) while determining the relationship between two factors which might be influenced by this third factor. The correlation of the two variables contains common elements in addition to the factors being related. The relationship which is unique to the two variables is found when common influences are removed. The removal may be accomplished through experimental design by control of the common factor or factors or through the statistical process of partial correlation.

An illustration may serve to clarify the concept of partial correlation. The zero-order correlation between mental age and skeletal development of children six to sixteen years old is around .85. This is a very high relationship between measures of mental and physiological maturity. However, the chronological age of the children varied over most of the growth years; and, both mental age and skeletal development increase regularly with chronological age. Thus, age is a factor that enhances the magnitude of the correspondence between mental age and skeletal development. With age held constant, the correlation between these tests is low; actually, it is insignificant. Age can be held constant by correlating the two variables for children of the same age. However, the partial-correlation technique accomplishes the same result; with age partialled out, the resultant correlation is comparable to the zero-order correlation when children of the same age are subjects.

FIRST-ORDER PARTIAL CORRELATION

In first-order partial correlation, three variables are involved, one of which is held constant. These variables are numbered 1, 2, and 3; formerly, in zero-order correlation, the variables were designated as x and y. Thus, r_{12} indicates the zero order correlation between variables 1 and 2. The symbol for a partial correlation between variables 1 and 2 with 3 held constant is $r_{12.3}$. Three partial correlations can be obtained for these three variables. The formulas are:

$$r_{12.3} = \frac{r_{12} - r_{13}r_{23}}{\sqrt{1 - r_{13}^2}\,\sqrt{1 - r_{23}^2}} \tag{3.1}$$

$$r_{13.2} = \frac{r_{13} - r_{12}r_{23}}{\sqrt{1 - r_{12}^2}\,\sqrt{1 - r_{23}^2}} \tag{3.2}$$

$$r_{23.1} = \frac{r_{23} - r_{12}r_{13}}{\sqrt{1 - r_{12}^2}\,\sqrt{1 - r_{13}^2}} \tag{3.3}$$

The above formulas for partial correlations can be simplified a bit by combining the expressions in the denominators. For example, the denominator for formula 3.1 can be written: $\sqrt{(1 - r_{13}^2)(1 - r_{23}^2)}$. The form of the numbered formulas, however, will be used in this presentation, as the value for $\sqrt{1 - r^2}$ can be obtained directly from Table D in the appendix. To illustrate: if $r = .67$, $\sqrt{1 - .67^2} = .742$ from the table.

However, all three partial correlations may not be wanted in a given study; the purpose of the study will determine the ones desired. Furthermore, in some instances, partial correlations may not make sense or may be plain ridiculous in their implications. Such situations will be found in the following example from correlations reported by Bovard, Cozens, and Hagman.[1]

---

[1] John F. Bovard, Frederick W. Cozens, and Patricia E. Hagman, *Tests and Measurements in Physical Education* (Philadelphia, Penn.: W. B. Saunders Company, 1949), p. 375.

Variables	Zero-order Correlations
1 Shot-put distance	$r_{12} = .520$
2 Weight	$r_{13} = .395$
3 Height	$r_{23} = .583$

Two partial correlations would have meaning for the investigator, as follows:

Formula 3.1: $r_{12.3} = \dfrac{.520 - (.395)(.583)}{\sqrt{1 - .395^2}\ \sqrt{1 - .583^2}} = .389$

In this instance, the zero-order correlation between shot-put ability and weight is .520. When the height of the performers is partialled out, the correlation declines to .389. Thus, the height of the shot putters has some value unaccounted for by weight.

Formula 3.2: $r_{13.2} = \dfrac{.395 - (.520)(.583)}{\sqrt{1 - .520^2}\ \sqrt{1 - .583^2}} = .132$

Here, the zero-order correlation between shot-put performance and height was .395. The partialling out of weight reduced the correlation to .132.

The final first-order partial correlation, $r_{23.1}$, does not make sense. This correlation would give the relationship between height and weight when all subjects could put the shot the same distance.

An illustration of a first-order problem in which the investigator would be interested in only one of the partial correlation is taken from a study by Carter.[2] As a phase of his study, he related age and weight to Rogers' Strength Index for boys from nine to seventeen years of age. The essential correlational data were:

Variables	Zero-order Correlations
1. Strength Index	$r_{12} = .86$
2. Weight	$r_{13} = .86$
3. Age	$r_{23} = .82$

$$r_{12.3} = \frac{r_{12} - r_{13}r_{23}}{\sqrt{1 - r_{13}^2}\ \sqrt{1 - r_{23}^2}}$$

$$= \frac{.86 - (.86)(.82)}{\sqrt{1 - .86^2}\ \sqrt{1 - .82^2}} = .48$$

With age ranging over an inclusive span of nine years, the correlation

[2] Gavin H. Carter, "Reconstruction of the Rogers Strength and Physical Fitness Indices for Upper Elementary, Junior High, and Senior High School Boys," Microcard doctoral dissertation, University of Oregon, 1958.

between Strength Index and weight was .86. When age was held constant, the partial correlation was .48. As will be seen in the zero-order correlations, the partialled variable, age, correlated as high as did weight with Strength Index; also, it correlated nearly as high with weight. These circumstances are conducive to a much lower partial correlation ($r_{12.3}$) as compared with the corresponding zero-order correlation (r_{12}).

In the illustration given above, the partial correlations were lower than their corresponding zero-order correlations. Such is not always the case, as they could be the same or higher. To illustrate partial correlations that are higher than their zero-orders, data from a study of somatotype relationships by Munroe[3] will be given. The somatotype designates the physique type of an individual. With three numerals between 1 and 7 for each of three components the individual's physique type is described. The components are: *endomorphy*, defined as a preponderance of soft roundness throughout the various regions of the body with mass concentration in the center; *mesomorphy*, defined as heavy hard, and rectangular in form, with rugged, massive muscles and large, prominent bones; and *ectomorphy*, defined as a frail, delicate body structure, with thin segments antero-posteriorly. Each individual has a combination of these three components.

One might expect high correlations between endomorphy and weight and between ectomorphy and height. Such is not the case. The reason is that the somatotype components relate only to body form, not to body size; in other words, both big and little endomorphs and ectomorphs are found. However, partial correlations reveal the true relationships, as shown in the following tabulation in Munroe's study:

Somatotype Components	Zero-Order Correlations	Partial Correlations
1 Endomorphy	$r_{14} = $ .708	$r_{14.5} = $ .862
2 Mesomorphy	$r_{15} = $ .187	$r_{15.4} = $ −.709
3 Ectomorphy		

Experimental Variables		
	$r_{24} = $ .303	$r_{24.5} = $ .669
4 Weight	$r_{25} = $ −.188	$r_{25.4} = $ −.643
5 Height	$r_{34} = $ .505	$r_{34.5} = $ −.944
$r_{45} = $ .740	$r_{35} = $ .164	$r_{35.4} = $ .926

The zero-order correlations between height and the somatotype components were low, ranging from −.188 to .189. When weight was held constant, much higher partial correlations were obtained: −.709 for endomorphy,

[3] Richard A. Munroe, "Relationships Between Somatotype Components and Maturity, Structural, Strength, Muscular Endurance, and Motor Ability Measures of Twelve Year Old Boys," Microcard doctoral dissertation, University of Oregon, December 1964.

—.643 for mesomorphy, and .926 for ecotomorphy. When somatotype components were correlated with weight, the following respective zero-order and partial correlations with height held constant were found: for endomorphy, .708 and .862; for mesomorphy, .303 and .699; and for ectomorphy, .505 and —.944.

The use of a general formula will be introduced at this point. From a general formula, the specific partial-correlation formula for any combination of variables placed in any order can be written. General formulas will be used henceforth for the other multi-variable statistics in this chapter. The general formula for partial correlation follows:

$$r_{12.34\ldots n} = \frac{r_{12.34\ldots(n-1)} - r_{1n.34\ldots(n-1)}r_{2n.34\ldots(n-1)}}{\sqrt{1-r^2_{1n.34\ldots(n-1)}}\sqrt{1-r^2_{2n.24\ldots(n-1)}}} \qquad (3.4)$$

The numerals in this formula refer to the position or order of the numbered variables in a designated partial correlation. The symbol, n, refers to the last numeral in the partial order, regardless of the size of its number; and, $n-1$ refers to the next to the last numeral in the sequence. When the numerals are in consecutive 1-2-3 order, writing the specific formula is simpler. Thus, for a third-order partial correlation:

$$r_{12.345} = \frac{r_{12.34} - r_{15.34}r_{25.34}}{\sqrt{1-r^2_{15.34}}\sqrt{1-r^2_{25.34}}}$$

When the numerals are scrambled:

$$r_{35.164} = \frac{r_{35.16} - r_{34.16}r_{54.16}}{\sqrt{1-r^2_{34.16}}\sqrt{1-r^2_{54.16}}}$$

In this formula, the last partial r can also be written as $r_{45.16}$. The numerals on either side of the decimal can be re-arranged in any order without changing the answer.

As can be seen from the above, partial correlations of any order are computed from correlations of the immediately lower order. Thus, the third-order partials above require second-order partials; and the second-order partials need first-order partials; and the first-order partials are based on zero-order correlations.

Null Hypothesis. In interpreting the product-moment correlation in chapter 11 of *Research Processes in Physical Education, Recreation, and*

Health, it was shown that the distribution of r's of repeated samples from the same population conformed to normal probability only when the population r is zero; with a high population r, the distribution of sample r's is skewed and leptokurtic. The same situation prevails for partial correlations. So, the same adjustments made in interpreting the zero-order correlation apply to a partial correlation.

To determine the significance of a partial correlation, then, the null hypothesis is applied: The hypothesis is tested that the population partial correlation is in fact zero and any amount obtained from a sample is due to sampling error. As for product-moment correlations, partial correlations needed for significance at the .05 and .01 levels can be obtained from a table. Table E in the appendix provides these correlations plus those necessary for multiple correlations presented later in this chapter. For partial correlations, enter column 2; the amounts in this column are the same as in Table 19 of *Research Processes.* The only difference is in degrees of freedom; $df = N - m$, in which m is the number of variables in the partial correlation. Actually, this was done for the product-moment correlation as it has two variables, so $df = N - 2$.

To illustrate this procedure, reference is made to the above partial correlation of shot put distance. In this study: $r_{12.3} = .389$; $r_{13.2} = .132$; assume $N = 33$. The $df = N - m = 33 - 3 = 30$. Thus, enter column 2 and row 30 of Table E; partial correlations needed to reject the null hypothesis are .349 and .449 at the .05 and .01 levels. In this problem, therefore, the $r_{12.3}$ of .389 is significant at the .05 level; the $r_{13.2}$ of .132 is not significant.

Differences between Partial Correlations.   The significance of the difference between partial correlations can be tested in the same manner as for the difference between zero-order correlations explained in chapter 11 of *Research Processes.* The partial correlations are converted to Fisher z coefficients and the difference between the z-coefficient equivalents is tested for significance by application of the t ratio.

To illustrate this procedure, the differences between partial correlations of two groups of 207 subjects each will be used. The variable numbers and partial correlations are:

1 Endomorphy	$r_{14.5} = .86$
2 Mesomorphy	$r_{24.5} = .67$
4 Weight	$N = 207$
5 Height	

The partial correlations are converted to z coefficients by use of Table F in the appendix. Thus:

Partial Correlations	z Coefficients
.86	1.29
.67	.81
	$D_z =$ .48

The formula for the standard error of the difference between z coefficients is:

$$\sigma D_z = \sqrt{\frac{1}{N-m-1} + \frac{1}{N-m-1}} \qquad (3.5)$$

$$= \sqrt{\frac{1}{207-3-1} + \frac{1}{207-3-1}} = .10$$

$$t = \frac{D_z}{\sigma D_z} = \frac{.48}{.10} = 4.8$$

The t ratios needed for significance at the .05 and .01 levels are given in the last column of Table E; these values are the same as those appearing in Table 15 of *Research Processes*. Enter this table with:

$$df = (N_1 - m - 1) + (N_2 - m - 1)$$
$$\text{or} \quad = (207 - 3 - 1) + (207 - 3 - 1) = 406$$

From Table E, then, the t ratios required for significance at the .05 and .01 levels for $df = 406$ are 1.97 and 2.59. Thus, the t ratio of 4.8 for this problem denotes significance between the partial correlations beyond the .01 level.

LIMITATIONS

A number of limitations should be placed upon the use of partial correlations in research, as follows:

1. Valid relationships are possible from partial correlations only when data are linear. Linearity was discussed in *Research Processes* as essential for product-moment correlation. Inasmuch as partial correlation of all orders is computed basically from product-moment correlations, the same assumptions and requisites apply.

2. The investigator should still be cautious in interpreting cause and effect relationships. He may be more confident in identifying causative factors from partial than from zero-order correlation. However, the possibility continues that still unknown causes may be operating in the correlational situation.

3. A large number of subjects is most desirable to justify the use of partial correlation. When the number of subjects is large, the reliabilities of sample product-moment correlations are much greater (i.e., less subject to

sampling fluctuations) than when samples are small. For example, in a first-order partial correlation with all zero-order correlations equal to .80, the partial correlation is .44. By decreasing and increasing the first r in the numerator of the formula (r_{12} in formula 3.1) by .10 and keeping the other two correlations at .80, the partial r's are .17 and .72 respectively. The likelihood of such fluctuations by sampling error when the sample is large is slight, if not non-existent.

ILLUSTRATED PROBLEMS

The use of partial correlations may be observed in a study by Wilmore.[4] The relationship was studied between maximal oxygen intake (Max VO_2) and endurance capacity in a sample of 30 male subjects. The endurance test was given in terms of work output and riding time on a bicycle ergometer; in addition, each subject was given a densitometric estimation of lean body weight and percent fat. The correlation between Max VO_2 (liters/min.) and endurance capacity was .84; maximal oxygen uptake expressed in relation to body weight or lean body weight correlated low with endurance (.18). However, when the influences of body weight were held constant, the subsequent partial correlations between Max VO_2 (ml/kg./min and ml/LBW/min.) and endurance capacity improved to .78 and .64, respectively.

In an investigation of the relationship between skeletal age and other indicators of physical maturity to measures of muscular strength and motor performance, Rarick and Oyster[5] tested 48 second-grade boys. Maturity variables included skeletal age, chronological age, height, and weight; performance variables were eight muscular strength tests, standing broad jump, 30-yard dash, and a velocity baseball throw. Correlations between maturity and motor performance ranged from .21 to .74. However, when partial correlations were computed holding the various maturity factors constant, it was found that skeletal maturity did not account for a very large proportion (less than 9 percent) of the variance in strength and motor performance.

Partial Standard Deviation

In partial standard deviation, the variability of a given variable is determined when the variability influences introduced by other variables is eliminated. For example, the weight of boys varies more when the chronolog-

---

[4] Jack H. Wilmore, "Maximal Oxygen Intake and Its Relationship to Endurance Capacity on a Bicycle Ergometer," *Research Quarterly 40*, no. 1 (March 1969): 203.

[5] G. Lawrence Rarick and Nancy Oyster, "Physical Maturity, Muscular Strength, and Motor Performance of Young School-Age Boys," *Research Quarterly 35*, no. 4 (December 1964): 523.

ical ages of the subjects include several years than when age is limited to a single year. When boys' ages are from seven to seventeen years, the range of weights extends from a light seven-year-old to a heavy seventeen-year-old, estimated as 40 to 210, or 170 pounds; for a single year, say of twelve years, the range would be around 85 pounds, about one-half the larger range. The standard deviations are correspondingly affected. As for partial correlation, the effect of age can be held constant by confining the ages of the subjects to a single year, or less, or by computation of a partial standard deviation with age held constant.

A general formula for partial standard deviation is available, as follows:

$$\sigma_{1.234\ldots n} = \sigma_1 \sqrt{1 - r_{12}^2} \sqrt{1 - r_{13.2}^2} \sqrt{1 - r_{14.23}^2} \cdots \sqrt{1 - r_{1n.23\ldots(n-1)}^2}$$

$$(3.6)$$

The numerals in this general formula, as for partial correlation, refer to the position or order of the numbered variables in a designated partial standard deviation. When the numerals are in consecutive order, a third-order sigma is written:

$$\sigma_{1.234} = \sigma_1 \sqrt{1 - r_{12}^2} \sqrt{1 - r_{13.2}^2} \sqrt{1 - r_{14.23}^2}$$

When the numerals are scrambled:

$$\sigma_{5.316} = \sigma_5 \sqrt{1 - r_{53}^2} \sqrt{1 - r_{51.3}^2} \sqrt{1 - r_{56.31}^2}$$

or,

$$\sigma_{5.631} = \sigma_5 \sqrt{1 - r_{56}^2} \sqrt{1 - r_{53.6}^2} \sqrt{1 - r_{51.63}^2}$$

The numerals on the right side of the decimal may be placed in any order. Thus, the above two formulas will produce the same answer.

The orders for partial standard deviations start with the decimal, as the first variable in the sequence, σ_5 above, is the computed sigma. A first-order sigma is: $\sigma_{1.2} = \sigma_1 \sqrt{1 - r_{12}^2}$.

Illustration. To illustrate the use of partial standard deviation, data from the shot-put study reported by Bovard, Cozens, and Hagman, which illustrated partial correlations earlier in this chapter, will again be utilized. The numbered variables are: *1.* Shot-put distance. *2.* Weight. *3.* Height. The shot-put mean and standard deviation are 30.18 and 3.57 feet. Also: $r_{12} = .520$; $r_{13.2} = .132$.

$$\sigma_{1.23} = \sigma_1 \sqrt{1 - r_{12}^2} \sqrt{1 - r_{13.2}^2}$$
$$= 3.57 \sqrt{1 - .520^2} \sqrt{1 - .132^2} = 3.00 \text{ feet}$$

Thus, the shot-put standard deviation of 3.57 feet, as related to the mean of 30.18 feet, was reduced to 3.00 feet when the variability influences of weight and height are held constant.

Multiple Correlation

MEANING

A multiple correlation coefficient gives the correlation between a single variable and the combined effects of two or more variables. The correlation is obtained between a single test, or criterion, and a team of tests, two or more others taken simultaneously. In computing multiple correlation, some trait is being studied; the single test that represents this trait is known as the *dependent* variable, or criterion. The multiple tests with which it is correlated are known as the *independent* variables, sometimes called experimental variables.

A multiple correlations is not the sum of the zero-order correlations of the independent variables with the dependent variable. If such were the case, in many cases their addition would equal much more than 1.00. This is not the case, however, because the correlational influence of the independent variables is overlapping (i.e., they are intercorrelated) and so duplicate each other by varying degrees.

Multiple correlation is a most useful statistic; it permits the selection of the most valid battery of tests for forecasting a criterion. The chances of building up a multiple correlation by adding significant variables to the point where prediction is warranted are much better than when only a zero-order correlation is available. McCloy used this method for determining the importance of age, height, and weight upon athletic performance. Franzen depended upon this method to show the influence of social and economic factors on the health of children. Carter utilized multiple correlation to reduce the tests necessary for obtaining the Strength Index; without serious loss of validity; Hayman did likewise in selecting hand-wrist bones in the assessment of skeletal age.

COMPUTATION

The symbol for multiple correlation is R. Subscripts indicate the variables involved; the first subscript is the dependent variable and subsequent subscripts are the independent variables. Actually, the first two subscripts represent a zero-order correlation, so the other orders start after the second subscript. Thus, a second-order multiple correlation is designated as: $R_{1.234}$.

There are various ways of computing multiple correlations, all of which originate from zero-order correlations. Three computational methods will be described here; these are from partial standard deviations, from partial correlations, and directly from zero-order correlations.

Partial Standard Deviations.　The general formula for computing multiple correlations from partial standard deviations is as follows:

$$R_{1.23\ldots n} = 1 - \sqrt{1 - \frac{\sigma_{1.23\ldots n}^2}{\sigma_1^2}} \qquad (3.7)$$

As before for partial correlation and standard deviation, the arrangement of the subscripts is not the numbered variables but the position of the variables in the sequence. Thus:

$$R_{5.1739} = \sqrt{1 - \frac{\sigma_{5.1739}^2}{\sigma_5^2}}$$

This computation will be illustrated with the shot-put data utilized above for partial standard deviation. Thus:

Variables
1	Shot put	$r_{12} = .520$
2	Weight	$\sigma_1 = 3.57$ feet
3	Height	$\sigma_{1.23} = 3.00$ feet

$$R_{1.23} = \sqrt{1 - \frac{\sigma_{1.23}^2}{\sigma_1^2}} = \sqrt{1 - \frac{3.00^2}{3.57^2}} = .547$$

The multiple correlation of .547 was only a small amount higher than the zero-order correlation of .520 between shot-put distance and weight. Therefore, height adds little to the correlation already existing between weight and shot put performance.

Partial Correlations.　The general formula for computing multiple correlations from partial correlations is as follows:

$$R_{1(234\ldots n)} = \sqrt{1 - [(1 - r_{12}^2)(1 - r_{13.2}^2) \cdots (1 - r_{1n.23\ldots(n-1)}^2)]} \qquad (3.8)$$

As for the other general formulas, the order of subscripts refers to the position of the numbered variables in the sequence. Thus:

$$R_{5.1739} = \sqrt{1 - [(1 - r_{51}^2)(1 - r_{57.1}^2)(1 - r_{53.17}^2)(1 - r_{59.173}^2)]}$$

or

$$= \sqrt{1 - [(1 - r_{15}^2)(1 - r_{57.1}^2)(1 - r_{35.17}^2)(1 - r_{59.137}^2)]}$$

The rearrangement of the subscripts on either side of the decimal will not effect the computed multiple correlation.

In Carter's study[6] previously mentioned, the Physical Fitness Index for boys nine to eleven years of age was used as the dependent variable; the independent variables were the individual test items composing this test battery. To compute the highest first-order multiple correlation obtained, the following data are given:

Variables

1 Physical Fitness Index $r_{12} = .69$ $r_{13.2} = .72$
2 Leg Lift Strength $r_{13} = .56$
3 Number of Chins $r_{23} = .06$

$$R_{1.23} = \sqrt{1 - [(1 - r_{12}^2)(1 - r_{13.2}^2)]}$$
$$= \sqrt{1 - [(1 - .69^2)(1 - .72^2)]} = .864$$

The next variable added to the multiple correlation was lung capacity; however, it only raised the correlation slightly to .871. The multiple correlation of .864 was substantially higher than the highest zero-order correlation of .69.

Zero-Order Correlations. When only three variables are to be included in the multiple correlation, the computation can be made directly from the zero-order correlations. The formula is given below, together with an illustrated problem utilizing the above Physical Fitness Index data.

$$R_{1.23} = \sqrt{\frac{r_{12}^2 + r_{13}^2 - 2r_{12}r_{13}r_{23}}{1 - r_{23}^2}} \tag{3.9}$$

$$= \sqrt{\frac{.69^2 + .56^2 - 2(.69)(.56)(.06)}{1 - .06^2}} = .864$$

INTERPRETATIONS

Null Hypothesis. In determining the significance of a multiple correlation, the null hypothesis may be applied as was done for zero-order and partial correlations. As for the other correlations, also, Table E may be used for this purpose. The degrees of freedom are the same as for partial correlation: $N - m$. In the shot-put illustration above, $R_{1.23}$ was .547; suppose $N = 33$. Thus, $df = N - 3$, or $33 - 3 = 30$.

The change from partial correlation that is made for multiple correlation is to obtain the R's necessary for significance from the column representing the number of variables—3 in the illustration. Therefore, going down the column headed 3 to df of 30, correlations of .426 and .514 are needed for significance at the .05 and .01 levels. Thus, the R of .547 is significant at the .01 level. This procedure inflicts a more severe test of significance than if column

[6] Carter, "Reconstruction of the Rogers Strength and Physical Fitness Indices."

2 were utilized for all multiple correlations, as was done for zero-order and partial correlations. Had column 2 been used in this instance, the significant R's at the two levels would be .349 and .449.

Differences between Multiple Correlations. The significance between multiple correlations may be tested in the same manner as for the difference between partial correlations, when the number of variables in the two multiples are the same. Thus, the R to z-coefficient conversion is made; the σD_z is computed; and the difference between z equivalents is tested by use of the t ratio.

When the number of variables is not the same in the multiple correlations, an F test for such a difference may be applied. The formula is:

$$F = \frac{(R_1^2 - R_2^2)(N - m_1 - 1)}{(1 - R_1^2)(m_1 - m_2)} \tag{3.10}$$

The table of F (Table A in the appendix) is entered to determine the significance of the obtained F ratio. Two degrees of freedom are needed in order to enter this table, as follows:

Columns: $df = m_1 - m_2$
Rows: $df = N - m_1 - 1$

Suppose $R_{1.234}$ and $R_{1.23}$ are being compared, with an N of 30.

$$m_1 - m_2 = 4 - 3 = 1$$
$$N - m_1 - 1 = 30 - 4 - 1 = 25$$

Enter column 1 and row 25. The F ratios needed for significance are 4.24 and 7.77 at the .05 and .01 levels respectively.

Predictive Value. The predictive value of the multiple R may be estimated by the same kinds of procedures employed for zero-order r, as explained in *Research Processes*. The difference, of course, is in substituting R for r in the formula. These formulas are given here, illustrating with the above multiple correlation of .86 between the Physical Fitness Index and leg lift and chins.

1. *Coefficient of Forecasting Efficiency* (or Predictive index):

$$E = 1 - \sqrt{1 - R^2} \tag{3.11}$$

For the problem: $E = 1 - \sqrt{1 - .86^2} = .49$. The values for $\sqrt{1 - R^2}$ can be obtained from Table D.

This coefficient gives a rough percentage value of a prediction made from the correlation; and may be expressed as a percentage by multiplying E by 100. In this example, the R of .86 is 49 percent better than guessing when predicting the dependent variable. The *coefficient of alienation* may be used to indicate the absence of predictive value. The formula is: $k = 1 - E$.

2. *Coefficient of Multiple Determination:* $R^2 = .86^2 = .74$. This coefficient indicates the proportion of variance in the dependent variable (X_1) that is dependent upon, associated with, or predicted by the independent variables $(X_2, X_3,$ etc.) when proper regression weightings are applied. The *coefficient of multiple non-determination* may also be used: $K^2 = 1 - R^2$.

CONSIDERATIONS

A number of considerations should be mentioned in order to provide an adequate understanding of multiple correlation.

High Multiple Correlations.   High multiple correlations result when the correlations between independent variables are low, but their correlations with the dependent variable are high. In the multiple correlation of .864 for the Physical Fitness Index above, the independent variables correlated .06 and they both correlated moderately highly with the criterion; as a consequence, the multiple correlation was considerably higher than the highest zero-order correlation of .69 with the criterion. On the other hand, in the shot-put illustration, the independent variables correlated more highly (.583) than they did with the criterion; the consequence was only a slight increase for the multiple coefficient. Locating such variables, however, is not always simple, since tests which correlate highly with the criterion are apt to correlate well with each other.

Further, obtaining the best balance of low correlations between independent variables and high correlations with a criterion is difficult if a large number of variables are involved. In the day of the computer, a multiple correlation of all variables against a criterion is simple. However, the requirement of research problems may demand the selection of the minimum number of variables that will produce the highest R; invariably, three or four independent variables will suffice, so all the variables are not needed. For example, an investigator may be constructing a motor fitness test and has a criterion and 15 potentially useful test items. For his final test battery, he may want to select the minimum number of test items that adequately reflect the criterion by multiple correlation. The Wherry-Doolittle method is available for making these selections and will be presented in the next chapter.

Also, a "stepwise regression" computer program is available by which multiple correlations with a dependent variable can be computed for all combinations of independent variables up to a designated number, such as four or five. Invariably, as will be seen below, multiple correlations do not increase after four of the best combinations of independent variables are included. This program also computes the regression equation for each multiple correlation, as considered in the next chapter.

Correlations between Independent Variables. As indicated, the correlations between independent variables should be low to produce high multiple correlations. If the correlation between the two independent variables (r_{23}) is .00, for a first-order multiple correlation, the formula becomes:

$$R_{1.23} = \sqrt{r_{12}^2 + r_{13}^2} \qquad (3.11)$$

To illustrate, if r_{12} and r_{13} each equals .5:

$$R_{1.23} = \sqrt{.5^2 + .5^2} = .707$$

As r_{23} increases, $R_{1.23}$ decreases. For example, if r_{12} and r_{13} each equals .5 and $r_{23} = .9$, using formula 3.9, we get:

$$R_{1.23} = \sqrt{\frac{.5^2 + .5^2 - 2(.5)(.5)(.9)}{1 - .9^2}} = .51$$

This multiple correlation is only slightly higher than the zero-order correlations with the dependent variable.

Law of Diminishing Returns. Since the multiple correlation coefficient is not the simple sum of zero-order correlations of each of the independent variables with the dependent variable, but takes into consideration the inter-correlations among the several independent variables, the law of diminishing returns applies. This law states that when multiple correlations are developed, the greatest increase in the coefficient occurs with the first variable and the increases become smaller and smaller as new variables are added until no further increase occurs. For example, Schrodt[7] validated the Oregon Motor Fitness Test for high school girls. Her criterion was the sum of 12 test items; the multiple correlation developed as follows:

Variables	R	Increase
Hanging in arm-flexed position	.800	
Standing broad jump	.887	.087
Crossed-arm curl-ups	.925	.038
Knee push-ups	.952	.027

[7] P. Barbara Schrodt, "Objectivity and Validity of a Motor Fitness Test Battery for Girls in Senior High School," Microcard master's thesis, University of Oregon, 1958.

Frequently, the first increase in the multiple correlation is greater and the drop-off is faster.

Positive Relationship. The multiple correlation coefficient is always positive, ranging from .00 to 1.00. This result is obvious due to the squaring computations in the formulas. As a consequence, negative zero-order correlations with the criterion lose this identity. To illustrate such a situation: Clarke[8] correlated several independent variables with the standing broad jump distance of college men. The highest zero-order correlation with the jump was −.59 for abdominal fat; by adding hip extension strength, a multiple correlation of .66 was obtained. In describing the results, it is desirable to state that the multiple correlation was .66 with abdominal fat negatively related and hip extension strength positively related to standing broad jump distance.

Minimum Multiple Correlation. A multiple correlation will not be lower than the highest zero-order correlation with the dependent variable. It can be the same as the highest zero-order correlation with the criterion and, of course, it is usually higher.

Linear Relationship. Inasmuch as multiple correlation is usually computed from product-moment correlations, the assumptions for product-moment correlations must be met. The chief such assumption is that the correlational relationship must be linear.

Inflation. The multiple correlation coefficient computed from a sample tends to be slightly larger, i.e., somewhat inflated, than the R for the population from which the sample was drawn. This characteristic is especially true when N is small and m is large. This inflation is so small that it is usually ignored in research practice. However, Ezekiel has proposed the following "shrinkage" formula to correct for this situation:

$$_cR = \sqrt{1 - \left[(1 - R^2)\left(\frac{N-1}{N-m}\right)\right]} \tag{3.12}$$

To illustrate with Schrodt's multiple correlation above in which $R_{c.1234} = .952$; $N = 100$:

$$_cR = \sqrt{1 - \left[(1 - .952^2)\left(\frac{100-1}{100-5}\right)\right]} = .950$$

---

[8] H. Harrison Clarke, "Relationships of Strength and Anthropometric Measures to Physical Performances Involving the Trunk and Legs," *Research Quarterly 28*, no. 3 (October 1957): 223.

Suppression Variables. When a large number of variables is to be examined in relation to a multiple correlation, some investigators have eliminated those that did not correlate significantly with the criterion in order to reduce computational labor. On some occasions, this can be a risky practice, as such a variable may suppress the correlational effectiveness of other variables, that is, it may be a suppression variable. A variable may suppress in other independent variables whatever variance is not present in the criterion but may be in some other variable that does not otherwise correlate with the criterion.[9] The following example will illustrate this effect. Given: $r_{12} = .4$; $r_{13} = .0$; $r_{23} = .8$. Using formula 3.9:

$$R_{1.23} = \sqrt{\frac{.4^2 + .0^2 - 2(.4)(.0)(.8)}{1 - .8^2}} = .66$$

It must be admitted, however, that the occurrence of a variable that correlates .0 with X_1 and .8 with X_2, which in turn correlates .4 with X_1, is rare.

ILLUSTRATED PROBLEMS

With 79 college women as subjects, Sanborn and Wyrick[10] studied the relationships among standardized and modified balance tests, balance discrepancy scores, balance speed tests, and an Olympic Balance Beam Skill Test. For multiple correlations, the Olympic Beam performance test was the dependent variable and the balance variables were the independent variables. The product-moment correlation between the Olympic Beam test and modified sideward leap was .56; when standardized sideward leap was added, the multiple correlation was .81.

Servis and Frost[11] studied the personal and physical qualities of women which would most predict success in a professional preparation program of physical education. The criteria of success were academic index, a rating by the faculty, ratings by the student's peer group, and a composite of these three criteria. Predictive variables consisted of measures of physical fitness, general motor ability, temperament traits, mental ability, and values and interests. The single predictive variable yielding the highest relationship with success in the professional preparation program was the Rogers'

---

[9] For an explanation of suppression variables, see J. P. Guilford, *Fundamental Statistics in Psychology and Education*, 4th ed. (New York: McGraw-Hill Book Company, 1965), pp. 405–6.

[10] Carla Sanborn and Waneen Wyrick, "Prediction of Olympic Balance Beam Performance from Standardized and Modified Tests of Balance," *Research Quarterly 40*, no. 1 (March 1969): 174.

[11] Margery Servis and Reuben B. Frost, "Qualities Related to Success in Women's Physical Education Professional Preparation Program," *Research Quarterly 38*, no. 2 (May 1967): 283.

Physical Fitness Index for all criteria; the zero-order correlations ranged from .53 to .68. The highest multiple correlation obtained was .76; the dependent variable was a composite of the criteria and the independent variables were Physical Fitness Index, "active" temperament (Thurstone schedule), and mental ability (Otis).

Falls, Ismail, and MacLeod[12] investigated the validity of estimating maximal oxygen uptake from the AAHPER Youth Fitness Test Items, employing 87 male adult subjects. The dependent variables were gross O_2 uptake, O_2 uptake/kg. body weight, and O_2 uptake/kg. lean body weight. The highest multiple correlation was found between the AAHPER test and O_2 uptake/kg. body weight ($R = .760$). When the independent variables were employed in a regression analysis, it was determined that maximum O_2 uptake/kg. body weight could be determined by measuring pull-ups, 50-yard dash, shuttle run, and 600-yard run-walk.

[12] Harold B. Falls, A. H. Ismail, and D. F. MacLeod, "Estimation of Maximum Oxygen Uptake in Adults from AAHPER Youth Fitness Test Items," *Research Quarterly* 37, no. 2 (May 1966): 192.

4

PREDICTION AND THE WHERRY-DOOLITTLE METHOD

Meaning of Prediction

In prediction, results are anticipated beforehand. Usually, the anticipated results are not chance guesses but are based upon some known facts or relationships or are carefully conceived beliefs. The value of predictions is related to how much better they are than guessing. How frequently are they right? How frequently are they wrong? How close are they to actual results subsequently obtained?

Predictions of one sort or another are very commonplace in life. Examples are the teacher who drives his car to school in the morning with confidence that he will arrive safely, the broker who invests in the stock market in the belief that he will make a profit, the gambler who bets on a horse in the hope he will win, the Gallop poll that predicts the winner of a national presidential election, and the coach who names his starting line-up for a football game.

These predictions are not made in a vacuum; usually, they are not pure guesses. The teacher may always have driven to school safely, and so does not expect trouble. The broker utilizes a vast knowledge of the stock market and of individual stocks in particular to guide his investments. The gambler's bet is influenced by his knowledge of the past records of horses in a race, the condition of the track, the jockeys who are riding, and the like. The Gallop poll prediction is based on sampling the voting intentions of the American people. The football coach has watched and tried out his players under many conditions in forming his estimates of their abilities (and, if he is wrong, he can always substitute another player).

Colleges and universities predict when they admit freshmen to their institutions; the prediction is that those admitted will be successful academically and will eventually graduate. Typically, these predictions are based upon high school performances and various admissions tests. And, they are not always right, because the devices and instruments utilized do not have perfect validity in predicting college success. However, a constant effort is made by admissions offices and guidance personnel to improve admission procedures so that fewer and fewer wrong predictions are made. It is this attempt to objectify prediction—to the point where it may be incorporated into a statistical formula—that is the meaning and purpose of prediction in this chapter.

The statistical approach to prediction is through the use of regression equations. A better name for these would be "prediction" equations; however, the term "regression" has been in use for a long time, and is not likely to be changed at this late date. The concept of regression actually came before that of correlation, upon which it is now based. The term was first used by Sir Francis Galton in connection with his studies of heredity. He observed that the children of tall parents tended to be shorter and the children of short parents tended to be taller than their parents. This "regression" of the heights of offspring toward the mean of the population was called the *law of filial regression;* and the line portraying this relationship was called a *regression line*. The term "regression" is still used, although the original meaning of regressing to some stationary average does not apply.

Basically, the accuracy of predictions rests on the magnitude of the correlation. If the correlation is ± 1.00, prediction can be made with absolute certainty. If the correlation is .00, prediction is worthless, the same as random guessing. The higher the correlation the more confidence can be placed in predictions from it. Thus, the importance of a correlation is in terms of its predictive value. As was shown in chapter 11 of *Research Processes*, the predictive value of r does not improve on a linear scale but in a curvilinear manner. Thus, a very high correlation is needed before prediction can be made with reasonable assurance.

In this text, four regression equations will be presented as follows: regression lines on a scattergram, regression equation in deviation form, regression equation in score form, and regression equation in standard-score form. The first three of these equations will be presented for two-variable problems (r_{xy}). The last three methods will be shown in connection with multiple correlation.

Two-Variable Regression Equations

REGRESSION LINES

When the correlation between two variables is sufficiently high to warrant prediction, the simplest way to make the prediction is by use of regression lines drawn on a correlational scattergram. Once the slope of a regression line is computed and placed correctly on the scattergram, all predictions can be read directly from this graph.

Actually, two regression lines exist for a given correlation, as prediction can be made in one direction only and is not reversible, unless $r = \pm1.00$, in which case the two regression lines coincide. Frequently, the investigator is only interested in predicting in one direction, such as predicting X from Y in the computational illustration given below. In this instance, of course, a single regression line would be drawn on the scattergram.

To demonstrate the process of drawing regression lines on a scattergram, Figure 1 is presented. For this problem, a correlation of .87 was obtained between the number of times at bat and the number of hits for 102 major league baseball players. For purposes of simplification, only the scattergram form and the step intervals for the X and Y variables are given. The cells on the scattergram should be true squares for this purpose.

In this problem, it is quite likely that an investigator would be interested in predicting in only one direction. That is, he would want to predict the number of hits from the number of times at bat and not vice versa. However, for purposes of describing the calculations and drawing and using the regression lines, both lines will be included.

The essential data needed are r and the M's and σ'''s of the two variables. In the problem, the Y-variable is the number of times at bat and the X-variable is the number of hits. σ' is used in the formulas[1] rather than σ, inasmuch as the scattergram itself compensates for differences in the sizes of step intervals. In the scattergram, the interval for the Y-variable is 30 and the interval for the X-variable is 10, yet they encompass the same space. The M and σ for each variable are given in Figure 1. The necessary steps in drawing the regression lines follow.

1. Compute slopes of the regression lines. Two formulas are needed, one for each regression line. These formulas are:

a. To predict Y from X:

$$y = r\frac{\sigma'_y}{\sigma'_x}x \qquad (4.1)$$

b. To predict X from Y:

$$x = r\frac{\sigma'_x}{\sigma'_y}y \qquad (4.2)$$

The computations for this problem are given in the central column under the scattergram in Figure 1. The regression equations are:

$$y = .85x$$
$$x = .89y$$

[1] The standard deviation calculation without multiplying by the size of the interval.

REGRESSION LINES ON SCATTERGRAM
NUMBER OF TIMES AT BAT VS. NUMBER OF HITS
MAJOR LEAGUE BASEBALL PLAYERS

(*X*—Variable: Number of Hits)

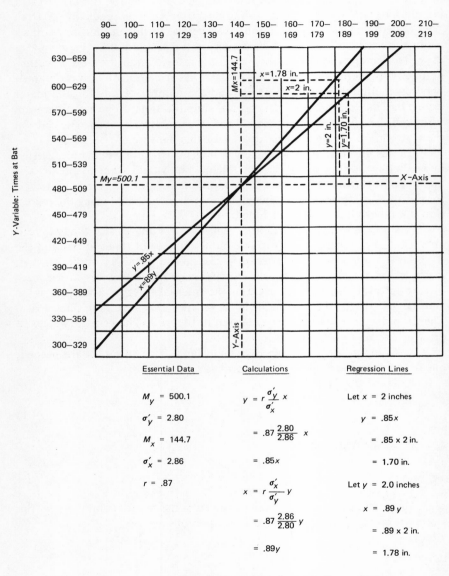

Essential Data	Calculations	Regression Lines
M_y = 500.1	$y = r \dfrac{\sigma'_y}{\sigma'_x} \, x$	Let x = 2 inches
σ'_y = 2.80		y = .85x
M_x = 144.7	$= .87 \dfrac{2.80}{2.86} \, x$	$= .85 \times 2$ in.
σ'_x = 2.86	$= .85x$	$= 1.70$ in.
r = .87	$x = r \dfrac{\sigma'_x}{\sigma'_y} \, y$	Let y = 2.0 inches
		x = .89 y
	$= .87 \dfrac{2.86}{2.80} \, y$	$= .89 \times 2$ in.
	$= .89y$	$= 1.78$ in.

Note: Original distances for plotting regression lines were 2 inches
When printed, these distances were reduced but remain proportionate.

2. Locate the point of origin. The point of origin for both regression lines is located at the central point in the scattergram where the means meet when plotted. The dashed lines on the scattergram represent the means of the two variables.

    a. For the X-variable, $M = 144.7$. This dashed line is drawn vertically down the Y-axis from the location of the mean in the X-distribution (about midway in the interval 140–149).

    b. For the Y-variable, $M = 500.1$. The dashed line is drawn horizontally across the X-axis from the location of the mean in the Y-distribution (about two-thirds up the interval 480–509).

    c. The point of origin is where these lines cross on the graph.

3. Draw the regression lines. As both regression lines will pass through the point of origin, a second point for each must be located. These points are located with a ruler using any convenient distances and substituting in the regression equations. This process is shown in the third column under the scattergram in Figure 1.

    a. For the regression line to predict Y from X, the equation is: $y = .85x$. If the distance for x is 2 inches, by use of the equation, the distance for y is $.85 \times 2'' = 1.70''$. These distances are measured on their respective axes from the point of origin. The second point for this regression line is located in the upper-right quadrant of the scattergram where these two distances meet, as shown. The regression line is drawn across the scattergram through this point and the point of origin.

    b. A similar procedure is followed for the regression line to predict X from Y. In this instance, however, the regression equation is $x = .89y$.

4. Make predictions from regression lines. The logical prediction in this problem, as already noted, is to predict the most likely number of hits from the number of times at bat (predict X from Y). For this purpose, the regression line $x = .89y$ is used. To illustrate the prediction process, let $Y = 420$. Locate Y in the Y distribution (lower limit of interval 420–449); cross horizontally from this point to the regression line; erect a perpendicular from this point to the X distribution; read off the value as 122. Thus, the most likely number of hits for 420 times at bat is 122.

To reverse this process and predict Y from X, let $X = 160$. Drop a vertical line from 160 to the regression line $y = .85x$; cross horizontally to the Y-distribution; read off the value as 539. Thus, the most likely number of times at bat for a player with 160 hits is 539.

It will be noted that the words "most likely" are used in indicating these predictions. Some such qualification of predictions is necessary since these predictions should not be considered exact. They are approximations and will always be so unless the correlation is ± 1.00. As pointed out earlier, of course, the higher the correlation the more reliable is the prediction. Also, the higher the correlation the closer will be the regression lines until they coincide at ± 1.00. The regression lines separate as the correlations become smaller until the mean lines are the regression lines at $r = .00$.

DEVIATION FORM

The regression equation in deviation form predicts scores from deviations from their means. Actually, the regression lines just explained are in deviation form also, inasmuch as the lines are related to the two means with point of origin where they intersect on the scattergram; and the slope of the line is determined from measurements made on the mean axes. However, the computation in regression form can be made directly without reference to a scattergram. The formulas for the two equations are:

$$y = r\frac{\sigma_y}{\sigma_x}x \qquad (4.3)$$

$$x = r\frac{\sigma_x}{\sigma_y}y \qquad (4.4)$$

The difference between these formulas and the ones used to compute the slope of the regression lines is that the full standard deviations are used (σ rather than σ').

For the baseball data utilized in predicting from regression lines, the regression equations in deviation form will be explained. The essential data are: $r = .87$; $M_y = 500.1$; $M_x = 144.7$; $\sigma_y = 84.0$; $\sigma_x = 28.6$.

1. To predict Y from X:

$$y = r\frac{\sigma_y}{\sigma_x}x = .87\frac{84.0}{28.6}x = 2.56x$$

The x equivalent for any X score is substituted in this equation. Thus, for $X = 160$:

$$x = X - M_x = 160 - 144.7 = 15.3$$
$$y = 2.56x$$
$$= 2.56 \times 15.3 = 39.2$$

As the X score of 160 is above its mean of 144.7, the y of 39.2 is above its mean. Therefore:

$$Y = 500.1 + 39.2 = 539.3$$

This prediction corresponds with the 539 predicted from the same X value of 160 when utilizing its regression line.

2. To predict X from Y:

$$x = r\frac{\sigma_x}{\sigma_y}y = .87\frac{28.6}{84.0}y = .3y$$

The y equivalent for any Y score is substituted in this equation. Thus, for $Y = 420$:

$$y = Y - M_y = 420 - 500.1 = -80.1$$
$$x = .3y$$
$$= .3\,(-80.1) = -24.03$$

As the Y score of 420 is below its mean of 500.1, the x of -24.03 is below mean (also, as shown by the minus sign). Therefore, X becomes:

$$144.7 - 24.03 = 120.7$$

This prediction is not exact with the regression line (122); the difference is due to overly generous rounding off of fractions in making the various computations.

SCORE FORM

The regression equation in score form makes possible predictions directly from raw scores (X and Y) without converting to deviations from the means (x and y). The equations in score form are derived from the deviation form formulas, as will be shown. The illustrated problem again utilizes the baseball data.

1. To predict Y from X:

     a. Deviation formula: $y = r\dfrac{\sigma_y}{\sigma_x}x$

     b. Derivation, substituting for y and x:

$$Y - M_y = r\frac{\sigma_y}{\sigma_x}(X - M_x)$$
$$Y = r\frac{\sigma_y}{\sigma_x}(X - M_x) + M_y$$

c. Computing the equation:

$$Y = .87 \frac{84.0}{28.6}(X - 144.7) + 500.1$$

$$= 2.56X + 129.7$$

To use the equation, substitute any X score. Thus, for $X = 160$:

$$Y = 2.56X + 129.7$$

$$Y = 2.56(160) + 129.7 = 539.3$$

2. To predict X from Y:

a. Deviation formula: $x = r\frac{\sigma_x}{\sigma_y}y$

b. Derivation, substituting for x and y:

$$X - M_x = r\frac{\sigma_x}{\sigma_y}(Y - M_y)$$

$$X = r\frac{\sigma_x}{\sigma_y}(Y - M_y) + M_x$$

c. Computing the equation:

$$X = .87\frac{28.6}{84.0}(Y - 500.1) + 144.7$$

$$= .3Y - 5.3$$

To use this equation, substitute any Y score. Thus, for $Y = 420$:

$$X = .3Y - 5.3$$

$$= .3(420) - 5.3 = 120.7$$

Usually, in practice, the constant at the end of the regression equation in score form is carried as a whole number. This practice would not be followed, however, if the range of scores were narrow and the fraction meaningful in predicting performance.

RELIABILITY OF PREDICTIONS

As indicated before, predictions from one variable to another cannot be made with absolute fidelity unless $r = \pm 1.00$. Thus, predictions based on correlations less than this amount must be approximations. They are subject to prediction errors greatly affected by the magnitude of r. This predictive error is known as the standard error of estimate (σ_{est}). The formulas for predictions based on the two regression equations[2] are:

$$\text{Prediction of } Y: \quad \sigma_{est\ y} = \sigma_y\sqrt{1 - r^2} \qquad (4.5)$$

$$\text{Prediction of } X: \quad \sigma_{est\ x} = \sigma_x\sqrt{1 - r^2} \qquad (4.6)$$

Table D in the appendix may be utilized to obtain $\sqrt{1 - r^2}$. Enter this table with r and read off the answer.

By use of these formulas, the reliabilities of predictions may be inferred in accordance with normal probability. The use of the formulas and interpretation of predictions utilizing them will be demonstrated with the baseball data.

Prediction of Y. In illustrating predictions from regression equations in the baseball problem, a Y score of 539 was predicted from an X score of 160. Thus, for a batter with 160 hits, his most likely number of times at bat is 539. How reliable, or accurate, is this prediction?

$$\sigma_{est\ y} = \sigma_y\sqrt{1 - r^2}$$
$$= 84.0\sqrt{1 - .87^2} = 41.2$$

To interpret in terms of normal probability, there are 68.26 chances in 100 that the player's actual number of times at bat is 539 ± 41, or between 498 and 580. At the .05 level, enter the right-hand column of Table E with $df = N - 1$ ($102 - 1 = 101$); the t necessary at this level is 1.98. So, the chances are 95 in 100 that the number of times at bat is $539 \pm 1.98 \times 41$, or between 458 and 620.

Prediction of X. To repeat the process with prediction of X: for a Y of 420, the X prediction was 121. Thus, for a player with 420 times at bat, his most likely number of hits is 121.

$$\sigma_{est\ x} = \sigma_x\sqrt{1 - r^2}$$
$$= 28.6\sqrt{1 - .87^2} = 14.0$$

To interpret: There are 68.26 chances in 100 that the player's actual number of hits is 121 ± 14, or between 107 and 135. At the .01 level, utilizing Table E again, the t necessary is 2.63. So, the chances are 99 in 100 that the number of hits is $121 \pm 2.63 \times 14$, or between 84 and 158.

---

[2] These formulas are the same as for partial standard deviations as shown in Chapter 3.

As can be readily seen, the magnitude of r has a great influence on the reliability of predictions. In the predictions above, the amount of error is large, even with an r of .87. The illustrations serve to stress the need for correlations approaching ± 1.00 (.95 and higher) before sufficient confidence can be placed on the accuracy of predictions. This observation will be further supported in the next section.

To illustrate further the effect of r on reliability prediction, consider r's of 1.00 and .00. Substituting each of these in the $\sigma_{est\ x}$ formula above:

$$\sigma_{est\ x} = \sigma_x\sqrt{1 - r^2}$$
$$= 28.6\sqrt{1 - 1.00^2} = .00$$
$$= 28.6\sqrt{1 - .00^2} = 28.6$$

Thus, when $r = 1.00$, no error is found for the prediction; when $r = .00$, the σ_{est} is the same as σ. Even with an r or .99, the σ_{est} is:

$$\sigma_{est} = 28.6\sqrt{1 - .99^2} = 4.0$$

The standard deviations, of course, also affect the predictive error; the larger the σ, the larger is the σ_{est} for a given r. This observation underlies the fact that prediction must necessarily be grosser when distributions are extensive than when the range of scores is narrow. However, this situation is relative to the distribution of scores since σ represents their variability.

Multiple Regression Equations

Regression equations based upon zero-order correlations were presented in the preceding section of this chapter. These procedures will be extended here to multiple regression equations based upon multiple correlations. Three equation forms—deviation, score, and standard score—will be presented.

The starting point for any regression equation is the correlation, zero-order or multiple, upon which it is based. In this instance, a multiple regression equation should be computed only if the multiple correlation is sufficiently high to warrant prediction from it. Then, the correlation identifies the independent variables to be included and their order in the regression equation.

DEVIATION FORM

While the regression equation in deviation form is seldom used in practice because of cumbersome manipulation, understanding it is necessary in order to use the common regression equation in score form. The general formula utilizes score weights, which also require a general formula. Actually, score weights were used, although not so designated, in the regression equations based on two variables. Two regression equations in deviation form were expressed in formulas 4.3 and 4.4, as follows:

$$x = r\frac{\sigma_x}{\sigma_y}y; \qquad y = r\frac{\sigma_y}{\sigma_x}x$$

The expressions $r(\sigma_x/\sigma_y)$ and $r(\sigma_y/\sigma_x)$ are score weights. Here, they will be given as partial regression (b) coefficients.

The general formula for multiple regression equation in deviation form is:

$$X_1 - b_{12.34...n}x_2 + b_{13.24...n}x_3 + \cdots + b_{1n.23...(n-1)}x_n \qquad (4.7)$$

To illustrate for an expression of the general formula for $R_{c.157}$:

$$x_c = b_{c1.57}x_1 + b_{c5.17}x_5 + b_{c7.15}x_7$$

In deviation form, of course: $x_c = X_c - M_c$; $x_1 = X_1 - M_1$; $x_5 = X_5 - M_5$; and $x_7 = X_7 - M_7$. Thus, in the use of this equation, all raw (X) scores must be related to their respective means. The use of this formula will not be demonstrated further here, but will be related to the score form equation to follow.

SCORE FORM

The multiple regression equation in score form permits prediction of the dependent variable directly from the (X) scores of the independent variables. The general formula is:

$$X_1 = b_{12.34...n}X_2 + b_{13.24...n}X_3 + \cdots + b_{1n.23...(n-1)}X_n + K \qquad (4.8)$$

As can be seen, this general formula is similar to the one for the regression equation in deviation form; the b weights are the same, but X is substituted for x and a constant (K) appears at the end.

Before this general formula can be used, the b weights must be computed. The general formula for their computation is:

$$b_{12.34...n} = r_{12.34...n}\frac{\sigma_{1.234...n}}{\sigma_{2.134...n}} \qquad (4.9)$$

The expression of this formula for $b_{25.689}$ is:

$$b_{25.689} = r_{25.689}\frac{\sigma_{2.5689}}{\sigma_{5.2689}}$$

To illustrate the computation of a multiple regression equation in score form: 100 boys 15 to 17 years of age were administered the Rogers' Strength Index battery. For this problem, the Strength Index is the dependent variable and leg-lift strength and arm-strength score are the independent variables; the multiple correlation was .978. The essential statistics for computing the multiple regression equation are:

Variables			
1. Strength Index	$M_1 = 2908.6$	$\sigma_1 = 401.1$	$r_{12} = .875$
2. Leg-lift strength	$M_2 = 1438.1$	$\sigma_2 = 280.6$	$r_{13} = .509$
3. Arm-strength score	$M_3 = 525.3$	$\sigma_3 = 151.9$	$r_{23} = .084$
$r_{12.3} = .970$	$r_{13.2} = .901$	$r_{23.1} = -.864$	
$\sigma_{1.23} = 84.6$	$\sigma_{2.13} = 67.4$	$\sigma_{3.12} = 65.6$	

The steps to be followed are:

1. Establish regression-equation formula in score form from the multiple correlation of $R_{1.23} = .978$, utilizing general formula 4.8:

$$X_1 = b_{12.3}X_2 + b_{13.2}X_3 + K$$

2. Establish and compute the two partial-regression score weights needed by use of general formula 4.9:

$$b_{12.3} = r_{12.3}\frac{\sigma_{1.23}}{\sigma_{2.13}} = .970\frac{84.6}{67.4} = 1.21$$

$$b_{13.2} = r_{13.2}\frac{\sigma_{1.23}}{\sigma_{3.12}} = .901\frac{84.6}{65.6} = 1.15$$

3. Substitute thus far in the score-form regression equation:

$$X_1 = 1.21X_2 + 1.15X_3 + K$$

4. Compute K, the constant derived when each X is related to its x equivalent. To demonstrate this process, the regression equation in deviation form is needed from general formula 4.7. Thus:

$$x_1 = b_{12.3}x_2 + b_{13.2}x_3$$

Substitute regression values, which are the same as for score form:

$$x_1 = 1.21x_2 + 1.15x_3$$

Substitute for x_1, x_2, and x_3:

$$X_1 - M_1 = 1.21(X_2 - M_2) + 1.15(X_3 - M_3)$$

Transfer $-M_1$ to the other side of the equation and substitute for the means:

$$X_1 = 1.21(X_2 - 1438.1) + 1.15(X_3 - 525.3) + 2908.6$$

Clear parentheses:

$$X_1 = 1.21X_2 - 1740.1 + 1.15X_3 - 604.1 + 2908.6$$

Collect values for K:

$$K = -1740.1 - 604.1 + 2908.6 = 564$$

Thus, the regression equation in score form is:

$$X_1 = 1.21X_2 + 1.15X_3 + 564$$

To illustrate the use of this regression equation, Steve has a leg lift (X_2) of 1500 and an arm strength score (X_3) of 300:

$$X_1 = 1.21(1500) + 1.15(300) + 564$$
$$= 1815 + 345 + 564 = 2724$$

Thus, Steve's predicted Strength Index (X_1) is 2724. When such a formula is used frequently, a table providing the multiplications for each independent variable can be constructed to expedite the calculations.[3]

Three Variable Equation. When multiple regression equations are to be computed from a first-order multiple correlation (three variables), the following formula utilizing zero-order, rather than partial, correlations may be used:

$$X_1 = \frac{\sigma_1(r_{12} - r_{13}r_{23})}{\sigma_2(1 - r_{23}^2)}X_2 + \frac{\sigma_1(r_{13} - r_{12}r_{23})}{\sigma_3(1 - r_{23}^2)}X_3 + K \qquad (4.10)$$

This is a general formula, so the numeral subscripts represent the order of the variables as established in the multiple correlation, as is true for other general formulas.

---

[3] This process is described in H. Harrison Clarke, *Application of Measurement to Health and Physical Education*, 4th ed. (Englewood Cliffs, N.J.: Prentice-Hall, Inc., 1967), p. 168.

The multiple regression equation may also be expressed in standard score form. Thus, the data are given as standard scores, which are standard deviation distances of scores from the mean, or: $Z = \dfrac{X - M}{\sigma}$. When all tests are standard scores, differences in test units as well as distances in variability become equal for all variables. Thus, all means are .00 and all standard deviations are 1.00. Usually, Z scales extend between ± 3.00.

In computing multiple regression equations in standard score form, beta (β) coefficients are used instead of score (b) coefficients. Inasmuch as the means are .00 and the standard deviations are 1.00, the constant K, found necessary in the score form formula, also equals .00, so is not needed. The general formula is:

$$Z_1 = \beta_{12.34\ldots n} Z_2 + \beta_{13.24\ldots n} Z_3 + \cdots + \beta_{1n.23\ldots(n-1)} Z_n \quad (4.11)$$

Again, the subscripts represent the order of the variables as established in the multiple correlation.

The beta coefficients can be computed from the b coefficients. The general formula is:

$$\beta_{12.34\ldots n} = b_{12.34\ldots n} \frac{\sigma_2}{\sigma_1} \quad (4.12)$$

The computation of regression equation in standard score form will be computed from the above problem for score form. The multiple correlation was: $R_{1.23} = .979$. The variables were: $X_1 =$ Strength Index; $X_2 =$ leg lift; $X_3 =$ arm strength score. The regression equation written from the general formula (4.11) is:

$$Z_1 = \beta_{12.3} z_2 + \beta_{13.2} Z_3$$

Two β coefficients are needed. The data necessary to compute these coefficients are available in the above score weight problem. Thus, the general formula for beta coefficients (4.12):

$$\beta_{12.3} = b_{12.3} \frac{\sigma_2}{\sigma_1} = 1.21 \frac{280.6}{401.1} = .85$$

$$\beta_{13.2} = b_{13.2} \frac{\sigma_3}{\sigma_1} = 1.15 \frac{151.9}{401.1} = .44$$

Therefore:

$$Z_1 = .85 Z_2 + .44 Z_3$$

To show the use of the formula, Greg's standard scores were: $Z_2 = 1.15; Z_3 = -.25$.

$$Z_1 = .85(1.15) + .44(-.25)$$
$$= .98 + (-.11) = .87$$

Thus, Greg's Strength Index in standard score form (Z_1) is .87; or, he is .87 standard deviation above the mean for this test.

The regression equation in standard score form involves a less easily understood, and perhaps awkward, concept than the more direct equation in score form. However, it has the distinct advantage of indicating the relative contribution of each independent variable in the prediction of the dependent variable. In the illustration, the ratio of beta weights is .85:44, or approximately 2:1. Thus, for the prediction of Strength Index, leg lift has twice the value of the arm strength score. In score form, the actual weightings of the variables are obscured by their respective shares in the constant, K.

Multiple correlations may be obtained from beta coefficients, utilizing the following general formula:

$$R^2_{1.234...n} = \beta_{12.34...n}r_{12} + \beta_{13.24...n}r_{13} + \cdots + \beta_{1n.23...(n-1)}r_{1n} \quad (4.13)$$

Thus, in this problem:

$$R^2 = \beta_{12.3}r_{12} + \beta_{13.2}r_{13}$$
$$= (.85)(.88) + (.44)(.51) = .9724$$
$$R = \sqrt{R^2} = \sqrt{.9724} = .98$$

The original multiple correlation for this problem was .98.

STANDARD ERROR OF ESTIMATE

Unless $R = 1.00$, some error is inevitable in any prediction from a regression equation. As has been shown before, the higher the correlation the less is this error. A standard error of estimate is available to indicate the amount of potential error. Actually, the standard error of estimate is the same as the partial standard deviation. Thus, the general formula is:

$$\sigma_{est\ 1} = \sigma_{1.23...n} \quad (4.14)$$

Applying this formula to the Strength Index problem:

$$\sigma_{est\ 1} = \sigma_{1.23} = 84.6$$

The use of the standard error of estimate is illustrated with Steve's above predicted index of 2724, assuming an N of 100. Enter the right-hand column of Table B in the appendix with $df = N - 1$, or $100 - 1 = 99$. At the .05 level, $t = 1.98$. Thus, at this level, the chances are 95 in 100 that Steve's actual Strength Index lies between:

$$2724 \pm 1.98 \times 84.6$$

or,

$$2724 \pm 167$$

or,

$$2557 \text{ and } 2891$$

Again, the need for high correlations in prediction is demonstrated. Even with a correlation of .978, the potential error in prediction is sizeable. Of course, in this problem, sigma was especially large (401.1).

COMMENTS

1. As was true for product-moment correlations and the partial and multiple correlations based on them, a basic assumption for the use of the regression equations presented here is that the data are linear. Thus, the scores on a scattergram follow straight rather than curved regression lines; the straight regression line is the line of best fit, with the scores distributed fairly evenly on both sides of the line.

2. In this chapter, the need for high correlations in order to have confidence in predictions is applied to individuals. Thus, if Scott has certain scores on select independent variables, his performance on the dependent variable is predicted by use of the regression equation. For group prediction, however, the correlations do not need to be so high. An illustration of group prediction is the selection of students for college entrance: by this prediction, a percentage of entrees are expected to fail college work but the individuals who will do so are not identified. Another illustration is from life insurance statistics: a proportion of an age group is expected to die, but the names of those individuals are not specified.

Wherry-Doolittle Method of Multiple Correlation[4]

The investigator utilizing multiple correlation usually wishes to select the minimum number of experimental variables that will provide the highest multiple coefficient with a criterion; and he wants to select them in the

[4] W. H. Stead, et al., *Occupational Counseling Techniques* (New York: American Book Co., 1940), Appendix 5. Also described in Henry E. Garrett, *Statistics in Education and Psychology*, 6th ed. (New York: David McKay Company, Inc., 1966), chap. 16.

order of their contributions to the correlation. The general rule given in Chapter 3 for producing a high multiple correlation is to select the variable each time that has the best combination of a high correlation with the criterion and low correlations with the other independent variables. This rule can easily be applied, with a minimum of trial and error, when a small number of variables are involved, thus the computational methods so far considered will suffice.

However, if a large number of independent variables are present, balancing of high correlations with the criterion and low correlations with other variables is hopeless. For example, if 20 independent variables and a criterion are involved, a matrix of 210 zero-order correlations must be evaluated. Computers can be programmed to produce a multiple correlation with all 20 independent variables. However, this does not allow the selection of the minimum number of variables. Seldom will more than three or four independent variables be needed to reach the maximum multiple correlation. Also, if a multiple regression equation is to be computed and subsequently used, such an equation with a string of 20 variables would be impractical, if not ridiculous. A solution of this predicament is to program the computer to calculate multiple correlations for all combinations of variables up to four or five independent variables and for all orders; i.e., with four independent variables the orders are zero, first, second, and third (stepwise regression program).

The Wherry-Doolittle test-selection method of multiple correlation provides a process for solving the problem of variable selection. This method selects the variables in order of their importance; the multiple correlation is computed cumulatively after each variable is selected. When the multiple correlation fails to increase appreciably, the process stops. Check points are located in each round of the test selection so that the presence of errors (if made) is indicated. After the multiple correlation is completed, the process may be continued to compute a multiple regression equation.

The Wherry-Doolittle method of multiple correlation will be described here. The data are test scores obtained from 100 boys 15 to 17 years of age in the Medford, Oregon public schools. The criterion measure is the Strength Index; the independent variables are the various tests composing this battery. The zero-order intercorrelations for these tests appear in Table 4-1A. Four work tables are also needed. These should be set up as shown in Tables 4-1B to 4-1E. Table 4-1F will also be needed if regression equations are to be computed. The step by step computational process follows.

SELECTION OF FIRST VARIABLE

Table 4-1B: With signs reversed, enter the zero-order correlations of the independent variables with the criterion in the V_1 row (Table 4-1A).

TABLE 4-1

*Wherry-Doolittle Method of Multiple Correlation
for Strength Index and Battery Tests for 100 Medford, Oregon Boys,
15 to 17 Years of Age*

TABLE 4-1A

Intercorrelations

	1	2	3	4	5	6	7	8
C	.019	.227	.509	.406	.373	.875	.655	.441
1		.562	.545	−.051	−.083	−.227	.053	−.353
2			.773	−.168	−.144	−.081	.135	−.245
3				.057	.154	.084	.295	.080
4					.657	.325	.320	.351
5						.235	.285	.346
6							.459	.380
7								.128
M	6.8	14.4	525.3	122.8	113.6	1438.1	442.3	266.8
σ	3.0	5.2	151.9	15.3	16.0	280.6	74.9	37.7

For C: $M = 2908.6$; $\sigma = 401.1$

Key:

C. *Strength Index*
1. *Pull-ups*
2. *Bar Push-ups*
3. *Arm Strength Score*
4. *Right Grip*
5. *Left Grip*
6. *Leg Life*
7. *Back Lift*
8. *Lung Capacity*

TABLE 4-1B

	1	2	3	4	5	6	7	8
V_1	−.0190	−.2270	−.5090	−.4060	−.3730	−.8750	−.6550	−.4410
V_2	−.2176	−.2979	−.4355	−.1216	−.1674		−.2534	−.1085
V_3	.0299	.0441		−.1086	−.1085		−.1410	−.0874

TABLE 4-1C

	1	2	3	4	5	6	7	8
Z_1	1.000	1.000	1.000	1.000	1.000	1.000	1.000	1.000
Z_2	.9485	.9934	.9929	.8944	.9448		.7893	.8556
Z_3	.6280	.3809		.8935	.9266		.7231	.8533

Table 4-1C: Enter 1.000 under each variable in the Z_1 row.

Table 4-1D: In row 0, place 1.000 in column c and N in column d ($N = 100$ in this problem). The steps for row 1 are:

TABLE 4-1D

a	b	c	d	e	f	g	
m	$\dfrac{V_m^2}{Z_m}$	K^2	$\dfrac{N-1}{N-m}$	$\bar{K}_2$	$\bar{R}^2$	$\bar{R}$	Test No.
0		1.000	$N = 100$				
1	.7656	.2344	1.000	.2344	.7656	.8750	6
2	.1910	.0434	1.0102	.0438	.9562	.9779	3
3	.0275	.0159	1.0206	.0162	.9838	.9913	7

Note: The shrinkage formula is incorporated in this computation.

1. Select the test with the highest V_1^2/Z_1 quotient as the first selected test in the multiple correlation. This process is easy on this round as all Z entries are 1.000. Thus, the highest quotient is for Test 6, the highest zero-order correlation with the criterion. The quotient for Test 6: $-.8750^2/1.000 = .7656$. Enter this amount in column b.
2. Column c: Subtract .7656 from 1.000 = .2344.
3. Column d: $(N-1)/(N-m) = (100-1)/(100-1) = 1.000$. The m is found in column a, and is the number of variables in the correlation (only 1, the criterion, thus far.)[5]
4. Column e: Multiply .2344 by 1.000 = .2344.
5. Column f: Subtract .2344 from 1.000 = .7656.
6. Column g: Take square root of .7656 = .8750. In this instance, the zero-order correlation between the criterion and Test 6 is returned, as only these two variables are in the multiple correlation. This is a check point; if the amount is not the same, an error has been made.

SELECTION OF SECOND VARIABLE

Table 4-1E: The a_1 to c_1 steps for this table follow.

1. Row a_1: Leave blank.
2. Row b_1: Enter the zero-order correlations of the variables with the first selected test, Test 6 (Table 4-1A). For the first selected test (No. 6) entry, the correlational amount is 1.000. For the correlation with the criterion, reverse the sign. Add the row and enter the amount in the Check-Sum column; in this instance, the amount is 1.300.
3. Row c_1: Multiply each b_1 entry by the negative reciprocal of the b_1 entry for the first selected test. Inasmuch as the b_1 entry for Test 6 is 1.000, the negative reciprocal is -1.000. For this round, then, the procedure is merely to reverse the signs of the b_1 entries.

---

[5] Application of shrinkage formula.

TABLE 4-1E

	1	2	3	4	5	6	7	8	$-C$	Check Sum	Test No.
a_1	-.2270	-.0810	.0840	.3250	.2350	1.0000	.4590	.3800	-.8750	1.3000	6
b_1	.2270	.0810	-.0840	-.3250	-.2350	-1.0000	-.4590	-.3800	.8750	-1.3000	
c_1											
a_2	.5450	.7730	1.0000	.0570	.1540	.0840	.2950	.0800	-.5090	2.4790	3
b_2	.5641	.7798	.9929	.0297	.1343		.2564	.0481	-.4355	2.3698	
c_2	-.5682	-.7854	-1.0000	-.0299	-.1353		-.2582	-.0484	.4386	-2.3869	
a_3	.0520	.1350	.2950	.3200	.2850	.4590	1.0000	.1280	-.6550	2.0190	7
b_3	.0105	-.0291		.1631	.1424		.7231	-.0588	-.1410	.8104	
c_3	-.0145	.0402		-.2256	-.1969		-1.0000	.0813	.1950	-1.1207	

TABLE 4-1F

	6	3	7	$-c$
c_1	-1.0000	-.0840	-.4590	.8750
c_2		-1.0000	-.2582	.4386
c_3			-1.0000	.1950

Table 4-1B: Draw vertical line through balance of table for first selected test, Test 6. Each V_2 entry is calculated from the following formula:

$$V_2 = V_1 + b_1 \text{ (criterion)} \times c_1 \text{ (test)}$$

The b_1 and c_1 values are in Table 4-1E. To illustrate:

For Test 1: $V_2 = -.019 + (-.875)(.227) = -.2176$
For Test 7: $V_2 = -.655 + (-.875)(-.459) = -.2534$

Table 4-1C: Draw vertical line through balance of table for first selected test, Test 6. Each Z_2 entry is calculated from the following formula:

$$Z_2 = Z_1 + b_1 \text{ (test)} \times c_1 \text{ (test)}$$

For Test 1: $Z_2 = 1.000 + (-.227)(.227) = .9485$
For Test 7: $Z_2 = 1.000 + (.459)(-.459) = .7893$

Table 4-1D: In this table, the second selected test is chosen and the multiple correlation with its inclusion is calculated. The steps are:

1. Select the test with the highest V_2^2/Z_2 quotient. Several trials may be necessary to make this determination. In this instance, however, Test 3 has the highest quotient: $-.4335^2/.9929 = .1910$. Enter this amount in column b_1, row 2.
2. Column c: Subtract this amount from the row 1 entry. Thus, $.2344 - .1910 = .0434$.
3. Column d: For the shrinkage correlation, $(N-1)/(N-m) = (N-1)/(N-2) = 1.0102$.
4. Column e: Multiply $.0434$ by $1.0102 = .0438$.
5. Column f: Subtract $.0438$ from $1.000 = .9562$.
6. Column g: Take square root of $.9562 = .9779$.

Thus, the multiple correlation with two independent variables is: $R_{c.63} = .9779$. With a sizeable increase in the multiple correlation, from $.8750$ to $.9779$, the selection of a third independent variable may be worthwhile, so the process is continued.

SELECTION OF THIRD VARIABLE

Table 4-1E: The a_2 to c_2 steps for this table follow.
1. Row a_2: Enter the zero-order correlations of the variables with the second selected test, Test 3 (Table 4-1A). As before (b_1 row), the entry for the last selected test is 1.000 and the sign is reversed for the correlation with the criterion. Add the row and enter the amount in the Check-Sum column;

in this instance, the amount is 2.479. After entering all correlations, draw a vertical line through b_2 and c_2 for the first selected test, Test 6.

2. Row b_2: Each b_2 entry is calculated from the following formula:

$$b_2 = a_2 + b_1 \text{ (test)} \times c_1 \text{ (2nd selected test)}$$

For Test 1: $b_2 = .545 + (-.227)(-.084) = .5641$
For Test 7: $b_2 = .295 + (.459)(-.084) = .2564$
For Check Sum: $b_2 = 2.479 + (1.300)(-.084) = 2.3698$

There are three checks in the b_2 row, as follows:

a. The b_2 entry for the second selected test (Test 3) should equal the Z_2 entry for same test in Table 4-1C.
b. The b_2 entry in C column should equal the V_2 entry for the second selected test (Test 3) in Table 4-1B.
c. The entry in the Check-Sum column as calculated should equal the sum of all entries in the b_2 row.

3. Row c_2: Multiply each b_2 entry by the negative reciprocal of the b_2 entry for the second selected test. The b_2 entry for this test is .9929. Thus, the negative reciprocal is: $-1.000/.9929 = -1.0072$

For Test 1: $.5641 \times (-1.0072) = -.5682$
For Check Sum: $2.3698 \times (-1.0072) = -2.3869$

There are three checks in the c_2 row:

a. The c_2 entry for the second selected test (Test 3) should be 1.000.
b. The c_2 entry in the Check-Sum column, as calculated, should equal the sum of all entries in the c_2 row.
c. The product of b_2 and c_2 entries in criterion column should equal the quotient V_2^2/Z_2 in column b, row 2, Table 4-1D, signs disregarded. The product: $(.4355)(.4386) = .1910$.

Table 4-1B: Draw vertical line through balance of table for second selected test, Test 3. The V_3 entries are computed as for the V_2 entries, except that the subscripts are now 2 instead of 1. Thus, the formula is:

$$V_3 = V_2 + b_2 \text{ (criterion)} \times c_2 \text{ (test)}$$

For Test 1: $V_3 = -.2176 + (-.4355)(-.5682) = .0299$
For Test 7: $V_3 = -.2534 + (-.4355)(-.2582) = .1410$

Table 4-1C: Draw vertical line through balance of table for second selected test, Test 3. The Z_3 entries are computed as for the Z_2 entries, except the subscripts are now 2 instead of 1. Thus, the formula is:

$$Z_3 = Z_2 + b_2 \text{ (test)} \times c_2 \text{ (test)}$$

For Test 1: $Z_3 = .9485 + (.5641)(-.5682) = .6280$
For Test 7: $Z_3 = .7893 + (.2564)(-.2582) = .7231$

Table 4-1D: The third selected test is chosen in this table and the multiple correlation with its inclusion is calculated. The steps are:

1. Select the test with the highest V_3^2/Z_3 quotient. Several trials may be necessary as before. In this instance, Test 7 has the highest quotient: $-.1410^2/.7231 = .0275$. Enter this amount in column b, row 3.
2. Column c: Subtract this amount from the row 2 entry. Thus: $.0434 - .0275 = .0159$.
3. Column d: For the shrinkage correction: $(N - 1)/(N - m) = (N - 1)/(N - 3) = 1.0206$.
4. Column e: Multiply $.0159$ by $1.0206 = .0162$
5. Column f: Subtract $.0162$ from $1.000 = .9838$
6. Column g: Take square root of $.9838 = .9913$

Thus, the multiple correlation with three independent variables is: $R_{c.637} = .9913$.

CONTINUANCE OF THE PROCESS

Continuance of the multiple correlation computation is not necessary since the coefficient has reached .9913, which is about as high as it can be. Stopping the process would also have been feasible for lower correlations if the magnitude of the multiple correlation had failed to increase or increase appreciably.

In this illustration, however, the process through Table 4-1E will be shown for three reasons: (1) The computation of the b_3 row has an additional feature that should be explained. (2) The check points in this table can again be utilized. (3) Data from this table are needed in the computation of the multiple regression equation.

Table 4-1E: The a_3 to c_3 steps for this table follow.
1. Row a_3: Enter the zero-order correlations of the variables with the third selected test, Test 7 (Table 4-1A). Add the row and enter the amount in the Check-Sum column. After entering all correlations, draw vertical lines through b_3 and c_3 for the first and second selected tests, Tests 6 and 3.

2. Row b_3: Each b_3 entry is calculated from the following formula:

$$b_3 = a_3 + b_1 \text{ (test)} \times c_1 \text{ (3rd selected test)}$$
$$+ b_2 \text{ (test)} \times c_2 \text{ (3rd selected test)}$$

For Test 4: .3200 + (.3250)(−.4590) + (.0297)(−.2582) = .1631
For Check Sum: 2.0190 + (1.3000)(−.4590) + (2.3698)(−.2582) =
.8104

There are three checks in the b_3 row, as follows:

    a. The b_3 entry for the third selected test (Test 7) should equal the Z_3 entry for the same test in Table 4-1C.
    b. The b_3 entry in c column should equal the V_3 entry for the third selected test (Test 7).
    c. The entry in the Check-Sum column as calculated should equal the sum of all entries in the b_3 row.

3. Row c_3: Multiply each b_3 entry by the negative reciprocal of the b_3 entry for the third selected test (Test 7). The b_3 entry for this test is .7231. Thus, the negative reciprocal is: −1.0000/.7231 = −1.3829.

For Test 4: .1631(−1.3829) = −.2256
For Check Sum: .810(−1.3829) = −1.1207

There are three checks in the c_3 row, as follows:

    a. The c_3 entry for the third selected test (Test 7) should be 1.000.
    b. The c_3 entry in the Check-Sum column as calculated should equal the sum of all entries in the c_3 row.
    c. The product of b_3 and c_3 entries in criterion column should equal the quotient V_3^2/Z_3 in column b, row 3, Table 4-1D, signs disregarded. The product: .195 × .141 = .0275.

MULTIPLE REGRESSION EQUATION

If the multiple correlation is high enough to warrant prediction, the Wherry-Doolittle process can be continued into a multiple regression equation in standard score form. The procedures follow.

1. Construct Table 4-1F from Table 4-1E. To do so, draw off the c entries for the tests selected for the multiple correlation in the order in which they were selected and for the criterion.

When equated to zero, each row in the table is an equation defining the beta weights. For the three tests selected, the equations are:

$$-1.000\beta_6 - .0840\beta_3 - .4590\beta_7 + .8750 = 0$$
$$-1.0000\beta_3 - .2582\beta_7 + .4386 = 0$$
$$-1.0000\beta_7 + .1950 = 0$$

2. Solve the third equation:

$$-1.0000\beta_7 + .1950 = 0$$
$$\beta_7 = .1950$$

3. Solve the second equation:

$$-1.0000\beta_3 - .2582\beta_7 + .4386 = 0$$
$$-1.0000\beta_3 - .2582(.1950) + .4386 = 0$$
$$\beta_3 = .3883$$

4. Solve the first equation:

$$-1.0000\beta_6 - .0840\beta_3 - .4590\beta_7 + .8750 = 0$$
$$-1.0000\beta_6 - .0840(.3883) - .4590(.1950) + .8750 = 0$$
$$\beta_6 = .7728$$

5. The regression equation for predicting the criterion from the three selected tests is written in standard score form by means of the following formula:

$$\bar{Z}_c = \beta_6 Z_6 + \beta_3 Z_3 + \beta_7 Z_7$$

Substituting the values derived:

$$\bar{Z}_c = .7728 Z_6 + .3883 Z_3 + .1950 Z_7$$

6. The beta weights can be changed to score weights if the regression equation in score form is desired. The general formula is:

$$b_p = \frac{\sigma_c}{\sigma_p} p \tag{4.15}$$

in which, the subscript p represents the variable; and the subscript c represents the criterion. The standard deviations appear at the bottom of Table 4-1A. To make the transformations in this problem (carrying to two places only):

$$b_6 = \frac{\sigma_c}{\sigma_6} \beta_6 = \frac{401.10}{280.63}(.7728) = 1.10$$

$$b_3 = \frac{\sigma_c}{\sigma_3}\beta_3 = \frac{401.10}{151.91}(.3883) = 1.03$$

$$b_7 = \frac{\sigma_c}{\sigma_7}\beta_7 = \frac{401.10}{74.90}(.1950) = 1.04$$

7. The regression equation in score form is now written:

$$X_c = b_6X_6 + b_3X_3 + b_7X_7 + K$$

Substituting values from step 6:

$$X_c = 1.10X_6 + 1.03X_3 + 1.04X_7 + 326$$

The constant, K, is obtained in the same manner as described earlier in this chapter.

ILLUSTRATED PROBLEMS

Maglischo[6] studied the bases for cable-tension strength test norms separately for upper elementary, junior high, and senior high school girls. At each school level and all school levels combined, the strength criterion was the average of 25 cable-tension strength tests; the independent variables were 12 anthropometric and 23 indices derived from them. By Wherry-Doolittle method, the highest multiple correlations limited to two independent variables each were: upper elementary school, .822, with height–times–cube–root–of–weight and arm girth/thigh girth; junior high school, .784, with chest girth–times–standing–height and shoulder width; senior high school, .607, with arm girth and shoulder width/hip width. When all school levels were combined an R of .844 was obtained; the independent variables were age and weight.

A handball skill test was developed by Pennington, Day, Drowatzky, and Hansan[7] from a total of 17 strength, motor ability, and handball skill test items. The criterion was handball playing ability as determined from each subject's average score per game in tournament play. The highest correlation with the criterion was .711 for the service placement test. The highest multiple correlation, as determined by Wherry-Doolittle test selection method, was .802; the independent variables were service accuracy, total wall volley, and back-wall placement. The score-form regression equation was: Criterion = 1.37 (service placement) + 2.27 (total wall volley) + 1.59 (back-wall placement) + .29.

[6] Cheryl W. Maglischo, "Bases of Norms for Cable-Tension Strength Tests for Upper Elementary, Junior High, and Senior High School Girls," *Research Quarterly 39*, no. 3 (October 1968): 595.
[7] G. Gary Pennington, James A. P. Day, John N. Drowatzky, and John F. Hansan, "A Measure of Handball Ability," *Research Quarterly 35*, no. 3 (October 1964): 258.

Clarke and Degutis[8] examined the relationship between the standing broad jump, as a criterion of leg power, and 16 maturational, anthropometric, and strength characteristics of 81 twelve-year-old boys. Seven of the correlations with the jump, all experimental variables being strength tests, were significant at the .05 level; these correlations ranged between .26 and .47. The highest multiple correlation produced by application of the Wherry-Doolittle test selection method was .694 between the standing broad jump and the independent variables of elbow flexion strength, body weight, hip extension strength, ankle plantar flexion strength, and leg length. The authors concluded that leg power was in part dependent upon body size and muscular strength, but cautioned that predictability of the standing broad jump was somewhat limited, since the coefficient of multiple determination was only .482.

Stepwise Regression Computer Program

In Chapter 3, it was indicated that a "stepwise regression" computer program is available by which multiple correlations with a dependent variable can be computed for all combinations of independent variables up to a designated number. This program also provides regression equations for each multiple correlation thus produced. The following studies illustrate the use of this process.

Sinclair, Gary D., "Stability of Somatotype Components of Boys Twelve through Seventeen Years of Age and Their Relationships to Selected Physical and Motor Factors," Microcard Doctoral Dissertation, University of Oregon, 1969.

Ward, I. Barrymore, "Longitudinal Analyses of Skinfold Measures as Related to Selected Physical Tests for Boys Twelve through Seventeen Years of Age," Microcard Doctoral Dissertation, University of Oregon, 1970.

Wiren, Gary, "Human Factors Influencing the Golf Drive for Distance," Microcard Doctoral Dissertation, University of Oregon, 1968.

---

[8] H. Harrison Clarke and Ernest W. Degutis, "Relationships Between Standing Broad Jump and Various Maturational, Anthropometric, and Strength Tests of 12-Year-Old Boys," *Research Quarterly 35*, no. 3 (October 1964): 258.

5

SPECIAL CORRELATIONAL AND NONPARAMETRIC METHODS

In this chapter, several correlational methods and a number of nonparametric techniques are described.

Nonparametric Statistics

At the start, the nature of nonparametric statistics will be explained, since both parametric and nonparametric processes will be described without a clear separation in this chapter. The parametric statistics previously presented are appropriate when the form of the population distribution is normal. When this requirement is not met, the data are *nonparametric*, also called *distribution-free*. Some nonparametric statistics considered in *Research Processes* are the median, percentiles, and quartile deviation.

Research data may be in the form of interval, nominal, and ordinal scales. The interval scale, the one most commonly found, contains equal units, i.e., the interval 15–19 represents the same amount as the interval 45–49. The so-called nominal is actually not a scale, but involves simply classifying individuals into categories with no order implied; an example is grouping athletes into somatotype categories. The ordinal scale places the subjects into rank-order positions. The statistics previously presented are primarily based on interval scales.

Whether a statistic is parametric or not parametric is not related to the form of the scales but to the assumption of normality, e.g., whether the population from which the sample is drawn conforms to the normal probability curve. McNemar[1] goes further and states that the crucial question is whether the t and F tests follow their theoretical sampling distributions when the underlying scores are not on an interval scale. He points out that the

---

[1] Quinn McNemar, *Psychological Statistics*, 3rd ed. (New York: John Wiley & Sons, Inc., 1962), p. 375.

assumption of normality, upon which parametric tests are based, may be violated to a similar degree without ill effects on tests of significance. This observation was supported by Boneau,[2] who computed 1000 t's for the differences between sample means for each of 20 different combinations of conditions with regard to the size of samples, the shapes of distributions, and equality or inequality of population variances. The percentage of the t's reaching the .05 and .01 levels indicated that the disruption produced by violations of assumptions was not as serious as it was assumed to be.

Chi Square

Chi square (χ^2) is one of the most versatile of all the statistics available, since it may be used to test various hypotheses and is applicable to a variety of situations. Chi square constitutes a test of significance. It is a generalized expression between a theoretical and an actual distribution, i.e., an actual response as related to an expected response. It can be used with either parametric or nonparametric data.

The simplest applications of a chi-square test occur for those cases in which the subjects of the sample may be divided into two or more mutually exclusive categories. The observed frequencies which fall into the various categories are then tested to determine whether their divergence from theoretical frequencies is too great to have occurred by chance, or, conversely, whether the divergence is so small that it could reasonably be attributed to sampling error. The theoretical frequencies are derived on the basis of the hypothesis being tested.

The chi-square formula is:

$$\chi^2 = \Sigma \left[\frac{(f_o - f_e)^2}{f_e} \right] \tag{5.1}$$

In which:

f_o = frequency of occurrence as obtained
f_e = frequency of occurrence as indicated by some hypothesis

The use of chi square is illustrated below utilizing a number of situations that might be encountered.

EQUAL OCCURRENCE HYPOTHESIS

A community recreation director surveyed a random sample of 150 adults in his community to determine their hobby interests in order to help

---

[2] C. A. Boneau, "The Effects of Violations of Assumptions Underlying the t Test," *Psychological Bulletin 57* (1960): 49–64.

develop his schedule of classes. Their preferences were: 56, art; 45, music; and 49, drama. On the basis of the evidence, it might be assumed that art groups should be sheduled with greater frequency than the other two, and music groups with the least frequency. However, realizing the role that chance plays in the selection of a random sample, the differences in choices might conceivably be due to sampling, i.e., there might actually be no preference in the choice of hobby groups in the total population from which the sample was drawn. The equal occurrence hypothesis, that theoretically equal numbers would choose each hobby, would be tested. To apply the chi-square test (formula 4.1):

	Art	Music	Drama	Total
f_o	56	45	49	150
f_e	50	50	50	150
$f_o - f_e$	6	5	1	
$(f_o - f_e)^2$	36	25	1	
$\dfrac{(f_o - f_e)^2}{f_e}$	.72	.50	.02	
				$\chi^2 = 1.24$

The degrees of freedom are: $df = (r - 1)(c - 1)$, in which r and c refer to the number of rows and columns respectively. In this case:

$$df = (2 - 1)(3 - 1) = 2$$

Enter Table G in the appendix with 2 df. The columns in this table refer to levels of significance; for example, the .05 column gives the χ^2 necessary for significance at the .05 level for various degrees of freedom. With 2 df, the chi square needed for significance at this level is 5.99. Inasmuch as χ^2 in this illustration is 1.24, the null hypothesis is accepted. From the results of his survey, then, the recreation director would be justified in scheduling the three hobbies equally.

CONFORMANCE TO A NORM

Drowatzky and Madary[3] conducted a normative physical fitness survey of boys and girls in the Coos Bay, Oregon, public schools. One of the tests had norms based on a statewide sample; the authors of the survey wanted to know if their Coos Bay results conformed with state expectations. The f_e, then, was the frequencies as expected from the norms. They used

[3] John Drowatzky and Charles Madary, "Coos Bay Fitness Survey," Microcard Master's Thesis, University of Oregon, 1962.

quartile groupings, so the expected frequencies were one-fourth in each group. To illustrate the computation of χ^2 for 260 seventh grade boys:

	1st Quarter	2nd Quarter	3rd Quarter	4th Quarter	Total
f_o	85	57	60	58	260
f_e	65	65	65	65	260
$f_o - f_e$	20	8	5	7	
$(f_o - f_e)^2$	400	64	25	49	
$\dfrac{(f_o - f_e)^2}{f_e}$	6.15	.98	.38	.75	

$$\chi^2 = 8.26$$

The degrees of freedom are: $(r - 1)(c - 1) = (2 - 1)(4 - 1) = 3$. Entering Table G with 3 df, the necessary χ^2 at the .05 level is 7.82; at .02 level, the amount is 9.84. Thus, the null hypothesis in this problem would be rejected at the .05 level.

A feature of chi square, illustrated in this problem, is that the significance of a departure from the expected frequencies can be determined; if significant, however, it does not indicate the manner or direction of departure. In the illustration, the greatest departure from expectation was in the first quarter; 85 seventh grade boys fell in this quarter while the expectation according to the state norms was 65. Other deviations are possible and must be determined by inspecting the distribution. Other non-conformity possibilities are a bunching of scores toward the upper end or in the middle of the distribution. If scores are bunched in the middle, the means may be essentially the same, but the distributions are quite different.

CONTINGENCY TABLE

A further application of χ^2 can be made when one wishes to find the relationship between traits or attributes which are classified into two or more categories. In such instances, χ^2 is computed from a contingency table; independence values are computed for the expected frequencies.

For example, school health authorities investigated whether or not flavored milk would increase the consumption of milk in the school cafeteria. The choice and consumption of milk was checked for a period of time with four flavors made available: plain, chocolate, strawberry, and orange. The results are shown in Table 5-1. The null hypothesis tested is that no relationship exists between milk consumption and the flavor of the milk.

The independence values that compose the f_e in the contingency table are obtained by multiplying the frequencies of the rows and columns for a given cell and dividing this amount by N. For example, in the upper left-hand cell containing an f_o of 30, the column and row frequencies are 162 and 70 respectively and N equals 300. Thus: $(162)(70)/300 = 37.8$. The chi square for each cell is then computed from formula 5.1 in the usual manner (part B of the table).

TABLE 5-1

Chi-Square Test by Contingency Coefficient
for Flavor and Milk Consumption

Flavor	Consumed	Partially Consumed	Not Consumed	Flavor Reaction Total
Plain	30 (37.8)	18 (15.4)	22 (16.8)	70
Chocolate	45 (40.5)	15 (16.5)	15 (18.0)	75
Strawberry	48 (43.7)	16 (17.8)	17 (19.4)	81
Orange	39 (40.0)	17 (16.3)	18 (17.8)	74
Totals	162	66	72	300

A. Calculation of Independence Values (f_e):

$$\frac{162 \times 70}{300} = 37.8 \qquad \frac{66 \times 70}{300} = 15.4 \qquad \frac{72 \times 70}{300} = 16.8$$

$$\frac{162 \times 75}{300} = 40.5 \qquad \frac{66 \times 75}{300} = 16.5 \qquad \frac{72 \times 75}{300} = 18.0$$

$$\frac{162 \times 81}{300} = 43.7 \qquad \frac{66 \times 81}{300} = 17.8 \qquad \frac{72 \times 81}{300} = 19.4$$

$$\frac{162 \times 74}{300} = 40.0 \qquad \frac{66 \times 74}{300} = 16.3 \qquad \frac{72 \times 74}{300} = 17.8$$

B. Calculation of χ^2:

The regular formula (4.1) is applied to each of the twelve cells in the above frequency tabulation:

$$\frac{(30 - 37.8)^2}{37.8} = 1.61 \qquad \frac{(18 - 15.4)^2}{15.4} = .44 \qquad \frac{(22 - 16.8)^2}{16.8} = 1.61$$

$$\frac{(45 - 40.5)^2}{40.5} = .50 \qquad \frac{(15 - 16.5)^2}{16.5} = .14 \qquad \frac{(15 - 18.0)^2}{18.0} = .50$$

$$\frac{(48 - 43.7)^2}{43.7} = .42 \qquad \frac{(16 - 17.8)^2}{17.8} = .18 \qquad \frac{(17 - 19.4)^2}{19.4} = .30$$

$$\frac{(39 - 40.0)^2}{40.0} = .03 \qquad \frac{(17 - 16.3)^2}{16.3} = .05 \qquad \frac{(18 - 17.8)^2}{17.8} = .00$$

These values added: $\chi^2 = 5.78$

The chi square for this problem is 5.78. To determine significance between the obtained and expected frequencies, enter Table G with the usual degrees of freedom: $(c - 1)(r - 1) = (4 - 1)(3 - 1) = 6$. The chi square necessary for significance at the .05 level is 12.59. Therefore, the null hypothesis is accepted.

NORMAL PROBABILITY DISTRIBUTION

When the hypothesis asserts that the frequency of events follows a normal probability distribution, the expected frequencies must conform to a normal distribution for the same N, M and σ as the sample. The normal probability table is needed for this determination. Other statistics books should be consulted for this computation.

SMALL NUMBER OF FREQUENCIES

When table entries are fairly large, χ^2 gives an estimate of divergence from a given hypothesis which corresponds well with other measures of probability. However, it is not stable when df is 1, a 2×2 table, and any cell frequency is less than 10 (some authorities specify 5). In such cases, Yate's correction for continuity should be made. The formula for χ^2 with Yate's correction is:

$$\chi^2 = \sum \left[\frac{(|f_o - f_e| - .5)^2}{f_e} \right] \qquad (5.2)$$

Thus, after each subtraction of f_o and f_e, an additional deduction of .5 is made. Otherwise, the computations are alike.

Yate's correction is needed because chi square is based on frequencies which are whole numbers, thereby varying by discrete amounts. The chi-square table, however, is based on values from a continuous scale. When frequencies are large, this correction is slight and may be disregarded; when the frequencies are small, however, the correction is of some magnitude.

DISCUSSION

The sampling distributions of chi square appear in Table G of the appendix. These distributions vary depending on the degrees of freedom. The smaller the number of categories, the fewer the degrees of freedom, and the smaller the chi square for a given level of significance. For example, for 1 df from a 2×2 table, chi square at the .05 level is 3.84; for 4 df from a 3×3 table, chi square is 7.78—double the former amount—at this level. Thus, the investigator may find some advantage in not proliferating categories when chi square is to be utilized beyond the number essential.

The fundamental nature of chi square can be explained in its relation to Z, the standard score (or standard deviation distance of a score from its mean). For example, in a normal distribution, Z at the .05 level is 1.96; $Z^2 = 3.84$, which is the amount for the .05 level in Table G. This relationship holds true only for 1 df. Distributions of chi square are not normal. Of course, the distribution of Z is normal, but squaring Z to obtain chi square (with 1 df) results in all values being positive and in changing the shape of the distribution. For higher degrees of freedom, each chi square comes from summing the chi squares in a manner which will not be described here.

The versatility of chi square stems from its additive nature, which is made possible by the squaring of the deviations. Because of this, too, chi squares may be added. For example, chi squares are computed from 2×2 tables (1 df) for the same problem but at three separate times. These can be added and the combined chi square tested for significance; 1 df is also added each time, so the df becomes 3.

ILLUSTRATED PROBLEMS

As part of a study of the relationship scores on the Wear Aptitude Inventory and selected physical fitness items, Campbell[4] employed chi square in the analysis of data. Eighth grade boys from six junior high schools were randomly selected as subjects. A chi-square of 40.41, significant beyond .01 level, was obtained between the distribution of the Attitude Inventory scores and similar scores from previously published data. The chi square for the distribution of scores between the six schools also differed significantly, but was found to be due to one school; when these data were eliminated, the distribution of scores for the two groups was not appreciably different. No significant relationship was found to exist between attitudes toward physical education and the ability to perform selected tests of physical fitness.

In a study designed to isolate and identify varying concepts of the course "Physical Education" as perceived by teachers and students, Wilson[5] gathered data from 119 physical education college major students, 46 teachers, and 283 high school students. Content analysis focused on physical fitness, sports and games, total development, social adjustment, recreation, and enjoyment. Several chi square comparisons were made among groups, but only when college students and teachers were combined with the high school group did a significant difference result. Fifty-eight per cent of the college-teacher group gave "total development" as the purpose for physical education, while the students identified physical fitness and sports-games as the main purpose.

Rank-Difference Method of Correlation

The rank-difference method of correlation, also known as the rho coefficient (p), was developed by Spearman to correlate two variables when

[4] Donald E. Campbell, "Relationship Between Scores on the Wear Attitude Inventory and Selected Physical Fitness Scores," *Research Quarterly 40*, no. 3 (October 1969): 470.

[5] Clifford Wilson, "Diversities in Meanings of Physical Education," *Research Quarterly 40*, no. 1 (March 1969): 211.

the data are in rank order. In some problems, scoring the subjects by ranking them 1–2–3 in their performances is either the most convenient or the only way to evaluate them. For example, a sample of boys in football could be ranked on two skills, tackling ability and blocking ability, both of which are presently impossible to measure objectively. Rho presents a means of relating these skills by correlating their ranks.

The investigator could also take data that are in score form and convert them to ranks for correlation by this method. This procedure would be as satisfactory with a small number of subjects as the more laborious product-moment method. In addition, if there were pronounced gaps in the scores, ranking would eliminate their influence in the correlational situation, resulting in a smoothing effect.

Rho is a nonparametric statistic. Ranks take account only of the position of subjects or items in the series; no allowance is made for gaps or differences between adjacent scores. For example, individuals with scores of 70, 69, 63, and 50 on a test would be ranked 1, 2, 3, and 4, although the differences between two of the adjacent scores is only 1 while the differences between the others are 6 and 13.

To illustrate computation of the rho coefficient: A number of years ago, the physical education faculty at Springfield College developed a form for rating the value for physical education teachers of ten intercollegiate sports conducted by the college at the time. A sample of 1,000 physical education alumni were surveyed to determine the number coaching each of these sports. A rank-difference correlation was computed between the faculty ratings and the number of alumni coaching the sports. The correlational process is shown in Table 5-2. The formula for rho is:

$$\rho = 1 - \frac{6 \sum D^2}{N(N^2 - 1)} \tag{5.3}$$

in which D is the difference between the ranks.

As can be seen in the table, both the faculty rating (R_F) and the alumni coaches (R_C) were ranked with the highest as number 1. Then, the differences between the ranks (D) were determined. Actually, in this process, giving the negative signs is not necessary since this column is squared; however, if they are listed, a check on accuracy is possible, since the sum of this column will then be zero. Finally, the D^2 column is computed and added. Applying formula 5.3, rho equals .80.

In the illustration above, a tie in faculty ratings occurred for track and field and baseball, each receiving 78.0 points. These sports occupy the ranks of 3 and 4, so both rank positions are used by averaging them, giving each a rank of 3.5. The next sport, swimming, receives a rank of 5. If three sports had been tied, the three ranks would be averaged and this amount assigned to each. When ties exist, a correction is appropriate if rho is to approximate the

TABLE 5-2
Rank-Difference Correlation for
Faculty Ratings and Alumni Coaches of Sports

Sport	Faculty Rating	Alumni Coaches	R_F	R_C	D	D^2
Basketball	87.8	830	1	1	0	0
Football	81.9	606	2	4	−2	4
Track and Field	78.0	456	3.5	5	−1.5	2.25
Baseball	78.0	665	3.5	3	.5	.25
Swimming	74.9	403	5	6	−1	1
Soccer	70.9	306	6	7	−1	1
Tennis	69.7	669	7	2	5	25
Wrestling	69.0	79	8	8	0	0
Cross Country	64.6	26	9	9	0	0
LaCrosse	56.6	16	10	10	0	0
					0.0	33.50

$$\rho = 1 - \frac{6 \times 33.50}{10(10^2 - 1)} = .80$$

product-moment r.[6] However, the correction is small and may be safely disregarded when only an occasional tie exists, as in the illustrated problem.

No generally accepted formula exists for estimating the standard error of rho, so confidence levels cannot be determined. However, rho can be tested against the null hypothesis by means of Table E, as was done for product-moment correlation. Entering column 2 of this table with 8 df ($df = N - 2$, or $10 - 2 = 8$), a rho of .765 is needed for significance at the .01 level. Inasmuch as rho for this problem is .80, the null hypothesis may be rejected at this level.

The magnitude and significance of correlations computed by rho are comparable to those computed by r when the underlying assumptions for product-moment correlation are met. Hotelling and Pabst[7] have demonstrated that the efficiency of rank-difference correlation is 91 per cent when compared with product-moment correlation. To interpret: a rho with $N = 100$ is comparable to an r with $N = 91$.

Biserial Correlation

Biserial correlation was developed for situations where one of the variables is measured in the usual continuous manner and the other variable

---

[6] See Daniel Horn, "A Correction for the Effect of Tied Ranks on the Value of the Rank Difference Coefficient of Correction," *Journal of Educational Psychology 33*, no. 9 (December 1942): 686–90.

[7] H. Hotelling, and Margaret R. Pabst, "Rank Correlation and Tests of Significance Involving No Assumptions of Normality," *Annals of Mathematical Statistics 7* (1936): 29–43.

is a dichotomy, i.e., divided into two categories. Occasions exist where measurement of one variable on a continuous scale is not possible because of lack of adequate testing instruments or the situation is such as to preclude such measurement; in these cases the investigator may resort to classifying the subjects into two groups. The original use of biserial correlation was as an equivalent to the product-moment method. However, it can also be used for point distributions, as will be explained later.

PRODUCT-MOMENT EQUIVALENT

When utilized as an equivalent to the product-moment method, the assumptions for biserial correlation must coincide. Thus, both variables must in actuality be continuous in nature, although one of them is not so measured, and linearity of regression must prevail. Proof of the assumptions may not be available for the dichotomous variable, and recourse to rationalization is frequently necessary; this rationalization may be supported with what is known about the trait represented by the variable.

Illustrations may serve to clarify this situation. The dichotomous variables could be athlete-nonathelete, physically fit-unfit, liked-disliked, and pass-fail. From what is known about the traits, certainly athletic ability, physical fitness, peer status, and ability on a test are continuous, distribute normally, and conform to linear regression. Thus, athletic ability ranges from the most inept in motor skills to the champion athlete; physical fitness ranges in degree from the physical weakling to those with great physical strength and stamina; peer status extends from the thoroughly disliked to the highly popular; and ability as demonstrated on a test varies from the ignorant to the completely competent.

The formula for biserial correlation is based upon the principle that, for a zero correlation, no difference between the means on the continuous variable exists for the two categories of the dichotomous variable. The greater the difference between the means, the higher the correlation is; the difference between the means is kept relative by use of the standard deviation. The formula for biserial correlation r_b is:

$$r_b = \frac{M_p - M_q}{\sigma_t} \times \frac{pq}{u} \qquad (5.4)$$

in which,

    M_p = mean, 1st category.
    M_q = mean, 2nd category.
    σ_t = standard deviation, continuous variable.
    p = proportion of cases, 1st category.
    q = proportion of cases, 2nd category.
    u = height of ordinate in normal curve dividing p and q.

The computation of biserial correlation is shown in Table 5-3. The continuous variable consists of individual scores on one test; the dichotomous variable consists of pass-fail performances on a second test. The steps are:

1. Compute the means for the dichotomous categories: M_p for the pass group and M_q for the fail group. These means are 98.27 and 83.64, respectively.
2. Compute σ_t, the standard deviation for the total group; this amount is 17.68.
3. Compute the proportions for the dichotomous variables. Thus, $p = .65$ and $q = .35$.
4. Obtain u from Table 5-4, as the height of the ordinate where p and q meet in the normal curve. The failing group (q) includes the lower .35 and the passing group (p) encompasses the upper .65 of the normal curve area. The point where these two proportions meet is .15 from the mean ($.50 - .35 = .15$). Enter the table with .15 area from the mean; the u for this amount is .370.
5. Enter the values thus obtained in the formula; the biserial correlation is .51.

An alternate method of computing r_b is also shown in Table 5-3. The formula is:

$$r_b = \frac{M_p - M_t}{\sigma_t} \times \frac{p}{u} \qquad (5.5)$$

The same correlation of .51 is obtained.

SIGNIFICANCE

The null hypothesis may be applied to determine the significance of the biserial correlation. As for the product-moment correlation, the standard error of a biserial correlation of .00 is computed and multiplied by the appropriate t for df. The formula is:

$$\sigma_{r_b} = \frac{\sqrt{pq}}{u\sqrt{N}} \qquad (5.6)$$

Substituting in the formula with the values obtained in Table 5-3:

$$\sigma_{r_b} = \frac{\sqrt{(.65)(.35)}}{.37\sqrt{200}} = .09$$

This amount is multiplied by the t in the last column of Table B for $N - 2$

TABLE 5-3
Biserial Correlation for
Individual Test Scores vs Pass-Fail Performances

Scores	Pass Group f	d	fd	Fail Group f	d	fd	Both Groups (total) f	d	fd	fd²
130–139	5	4	20				5	4	20	80
120–129	7	3	21				7	3	21	63
110–119	21	2	42	3	3	9	24	2	48	96
100–109	26	1	26	7	2	14	33	1	33	33
90–99	30	0	0 $\;109$	16	1	16 $\;39$	46	0	0 $\;122$	0
80–89	27	−1	−27	21	0	0	48	−1	−48	48
70–79	10	−2	−20	11	−1	−11	21	−2	−42	84
60–69	3	−3	−9	4	−2	−8	7	−3	−21	63
50–59	1	−4	−4 $\;-60$	6	−3	−18	7	−4	−28	112
40–49				2	−4	−8 $\;-45$	2	−5	−10	50
N	130			70			200		−149	629
	$\Sigma fd = 49$			$\Sigma fd = -6$			$\Sigma fd = -27$			

$$M_p = 94.5 + \left(\frac{49}{130}\right)10 = 98.27$$

$$M_q = 84.5 + \left(\frac{-6}{70}\right)10 = 83.64$$

$$M_t = 94.5 + \left(\frac{-27}{200}\right)10 = 93.15$$

$$\sigma_t = 10\sqrt{\frac{629}{200} - \left(\frac{-27}{200}\right)^2} = 17.70$$

$$p = \frac{130}{200} = .65$$

$$q = \frac{70}{200} = .35$$

$$u = .37 \; \text{(Table 5-4)}$$

$$r_b = \frac{M_p - M_q}{\sigma_t} \times \frac{pq}{u} = \frac{98.27 - 83.64}{17.70} \times \frac{(.65)(.35)}{.37} = .51$$

Alternate Method

$$r_b = \frac{M_p - M_t}{\sigma_t} \times \frac{p}{u} = \frac{98.27 - 93.15}{17.70} \times \frac{.65}{.37} = .51$$

TABLE 5-4

Ordinates (u) *for Given Areas from the Mean of Normal Distribution with Total Area of 1.00*

Area from Mean	Ordinates (u)	Area from Mean	Ordinates (u)
.00	.399	.26	.311
.01	.399	.27	.304
.02	.398	.28	.296
.03	.398	.29	.288
.04	.397	.30	.280
.05	.396	.31	.271
.06	.394	.32	.262
.07	.393	.33	.253
.08	.391	.34	.243
.09	.389	.35	.233
.10	.386	.36	.223
.11	.384	.37	.212
.12	.381	.38	.200
.13	.378	.39	.188
.14	.374	.40	.176
.15	.370	.41	.162
.16	.366	.42	.149
.17	.362	.43	.134
.18	.358	.44	.119
.19	.353	.45	.103
.20	.348	.46	.086
.21	.342	.47	.068
.22	.337	.48	.048
.23	.331	.49	.027
.24	.324	.50	.000
.25	.318		

degrees of freedom. Thus:

$$.05 \text{ level:} \quad .09 \times 1.97 = .177$$
$$.01 \text{ level:} \quad .09 \times 2.60 = .234$$

Therefore, a biserial correlation of .234 is needed in order to reject the null hypothesis at the .01 level. For the illustrated problem, r_b was .51, so the null hypothesis is rejected with assurance.

The use of a table to determine significance, proper for the product-moment correlation, is not appropriate for biserial correlation; neither is the use of the r to Fister z coefficient transformation justified for this purpose. The reason that these methods are not appropriate is that the standard error of the biserial correlation is not fixed for a given N as is true for the standard error of the product-moment correlation of .00. The standard error of the biserial correlation changes with each different proportion of p and q. The standard error will be large when the dichotomies are extreme:

when, for example, $p = .90$ and $q = .10$. The smallest standard error results when the dichotomies are split evenly ($p = .50$; $q = .50$).

Another method of testing the significance of the biserial correlation presented in several statistics books is by use of the t ratio. First, the standard error of the obtained biserial coefficient is obtained. The formula and computations are:

$$\sigma_{r_b} = \frac{\frac{\sqrt{pq}}{u} - r_b^2}{\sqrt{N}}$$

$$= \frac{\frac{\sqrt{(.65)(.35)}}{.37} - .51^2}{\sqrt{200}} = .073 \tag{5.7}$$

The t ratio is:

$$t = \frac{r_b}{\sigma_{r_b}} = \frac{.51}{.073} = 7.00$$

Entering the last column of Table E with $df = N - 2$, or $200 - 2 = 198$, the t ratios necessary for significance are 1.97 and 2.60 at the .05 and .01 levels. The t ratio of 7.00 is well above 2.60, and so is significant beyond the .01 level.

POINT-BISERIAL CORRELATION

When the dichotomous variable in a correlation problem is a true dichotomy, the point-biserial correlation should be used. Examples of true dichotomies are teachers as men and women, workers as employed and unemployed, and students at a university from in-state and out-of-state. Although they do not represent entirely discrete categories, bimodal or other peculiar distributions are sufficiently discontinuous to warrant use of the point-biserial correlation.

The point-biserial correlation is occasionally used for some variables that are not fundamentally dichotomies and may even be normally distributed. A frequently encountered case in point is the true-false question on an objective written examination. The true-false question tests knowledge, and knowledge varies from absolute ignorance of the question to its complete mastery, well beyond just recognizing it as true or false. However, since such questions are limited to separating individuals into two groups and only gross predictions can be made from the responses, the point-biserial correlation is commonly used.

The formula for point-biserial correlation is as follows:

$$r_{p_b} = \frac{M_p - M_q}{\sigma_t} \times \sqrt{pq} \tag{5.8}$$

DISCUSSION

The biserial coefficient of correlation is essentially a product-moment r and will give a good estimate of it if the assumptions for r are satisfied. However, biserial r especially cannot be used in a regression equation, has a much larger standard error than r when categories are widely split, and does not permit a conversion to the Fisher z coefficient. The biserial r may exceed ± 1.00 if the dichotomous distribution is bimodal or seriously non-normal in other ways.

The methods described here for computing biserial correlation apply to distributions where the full range of scores is included. Upon occasion, the investigator may wish to apply this method of correlation when only the tails of the dichotomous distribution are used, such as the upper and lower 25 per cent, although the tails need not be even. When such widespread categories are used, other formulas are necessary.[8]

ILLUSTRATED POINT-BISERIAL PROBLEMS

The use of the point biserial correlation is provided in one of several experiments conducted by LaBarba.[9] Forty graduate students were divided into two groups of 20 subjects each; one group received tactile sensations and the other kinesthetic sensations involving a pattern of dots and dashes; the subjects' task was to reproduce the pattern. In addition, information was obtained on their sports participation in high school or college. A point biserial correlation coefficient of .048 was obtained between sports participation and kinesthetic sensitivity; the dichotomous variable was participation and nonparticipation in sports. The point-biserial correlation between sports history and tactile efficiency was .55. The lower correlation for the kinesthetic sense suggests that perhaps it was less susceptible to experimental effects, that the limits for developing and promoting this quality were lower and more restricted than the tactile sense.

Employing 633 fifth and sixth grade children as subjects, 20 per cent Negro and 80 per cent white, Ponthieux and Barker[10] examined the relationship between race and measures of physical fitness, as expressed by the AAHPER Youth Fitness Test. The point-biserial correlations between race (dichotomous variable) and each measure of physical fitness (continuous variable) ranged from −.40 to .10 for boys and −.38 to .55 for girls. The data were arranged in such a manner that a positive correlation would indicate a tendency for white children to excel, whereas a negative correlation would

[8] For example, see Charles C. Peters and Walter R. VanVoorhis, *Statistical Procedures and Their Mathematical Bases* (New York: McGraw-Hill Book Company, Inc., 1940), pp. 384–391.

[9] Richard C. LaBarba, "Differential Response Efficiency to Simple Kinesthetic and Tactile Stimuli," *Research Quarterly 38*, no. 3 (October 1967): 420.

[10] N. A. Ponthieux and D. G. Barker, "Relationships Between Race and Physical Fitness," *Research Quarterly 36*, no. 4 (December 1965): 468.

indicate better performance by Negro children. The Negro boys exceeded the white boys significantly in five of the seven components of physical fitness. The Negro girls surpassed the white girls on four measures; two other measures favored the white girls.

Tetrachoric Correlation

The tetrachoric r can be used when both variables are dichotomies. This correlational method imposes the same assumptions as those for the product-moment method, i.e., the data are continuous and linearly related; the two methods are therefore comparable when the assumptions are met. In tetrachoric correlation, a 2×2 or fourfold table is developed. The development of the dichotomous variable in biserial correlation applies to both dichotomies by this method of correlation, except that the point distribution does not apply.

COMPUTATION

The first step in obtaining the tetrachoric correlation (r_t) is to construct a fourfold table. Such a table is shown in Table 5-5. The subjects are 14-year-old boys who were scored pass and fail on chinning and bar dip tests; scoring 5 chins and 8 dips constituted passes on these tests.

TABLE 5-5
Tetrachoric Correlation for
Pass-Fail Scores on Chinning and Bar Dips Tests

		Chinning		
		Fail	Pass	Totals
Bar Dips	Pass	20 (B)	37 (A)	57 (P)
	Fail	34 (D)	9 (C)	43 (Q)
	Totals	54 (Q')	46 (P')	100

$$r_t = \cos \frac{180°\sqrt{BC}}{\sqrt{AD} + \sqrt{BC}}$$

$$= \cos \frac{180°\sqrt{(20)(9)}}{\sqrt{(34)(37)} + \sqrt{(20)(9)}}$$

$$= \cos 49°$$

Enter Table 5-6 with $\cos 49°$; $r_t = .656$.

The fourfold table resembles the scattergram utilized for the product-moment correlation by the grouped-data method, as divided into quadrants by the lines representing the assumed means. The four cells containing frequencies are designated by the letters A, B, C, and D, and the columns and rows are identified as P and Q and P' and Q' respectively. These designations are made for identifying the various frequencies in the formula.

Several methods exist for obtaining r_t. The full equation is algebraically complex and involves the solution of a quadratic equation raised to several powers. However, a good approximation of the tetrachoric r can be obtained by the cosine method, especially if the two variables are each divided close to their medians. The formula is:

$$r_t = \cos \frac{180°\sqrt{BC}}{\sqrt{AD} + \sqrt{BC}} \tag{5.9}$$

The computation by this method for the pass-fail data on the chinning and dipping tests appear in Table 5-5. Substitutions in the formula merely consist of the frequencies in the cells as indicated by the designated letter. The cosine is derived as degrees of an angle: 49° in this problem. The cosine is obtained from Table 5-6; this cosine constitutes r_t. For cos 49°, $r_t = .656$.

The cosine angle varies between 0°, when B or C or both is zero, to 180°, when either A or D or both is zero. In the first instance, when the angle is zero, r_t is 1.00; in the second instance, when the angle is 180°, r_t is -1.00. When the product BC equals AD, the angle is 90°, the cosine is zero, and r_t is .00. In using Table 5-6 for angles between 90° and 180°, deduct the angle obtained from 180°, find the cosine of this difference, and give it a negative sign.

SIGNIFICANCE

The formula for the standard error of r_t is complex and generally not used. A simple and satisfactory procedure for determining the significance of r_t is to apply the null hypothesis. As before, this process consists of determining the magnitude of the correlation necessary for significance at a given level; the standard error for an r_t of .00 is computed and multiplied by the appropriate t. The formula is:

$$\sigma_{r_t} = \sqrt{\frac{pqp'q'}{uu'\sqrt{N}}} \tag{5.10}$$

The designations p, q, p', and q' in the formula refer to the proportions of P, Q, P', and Q'. Thus, in the problem:

$$p = \frac{P}{N} = \frac{57}{100} = .57 \qquad\qquad p' = \frac{46}{100} = .46$$

TABLE 5-6

Values of r_t for Cosine of an Angle

Angle (in degrees)	Cosine	Angle (in degrees)	Cosine	Angle (in degrees)	Cosine
0	1.000	37	.799	62	.469
5	.996	38	.788	63	.454
10	.985	39	.777	64	.438
15	.966	40	.766	65	.423
16	.961	41	.755	66	.407
17	.956	42	.743	67	.391
18	.951	43	.731	68	.375
19	.946	44	.719	69	.358
20	.940	45	.707	70	.342
21	.934	46	.695	71	.326
22	.927	47	.682	72	.309
23	.921	48	.669	73	.292
24	.914	49	.656	74	.276
25	.906	50	.643	75	.259
26	.899	51	.629	76	.242
27	.891	52	.616	77	.225
28	.883	53	.602	78	.208
29	.875	54	.588	79	.191
30	.866	55	.574	80	.174
31	.857	56	.559	81	.156
32	.848	57	.545	82	.139
33	.839	58	.530	83	.122
34	.829	59	.515	84	.105
35	.819	60	.500	85	.087
36	.809	61	485	90	.000

$$q = \frac{Q}{N} = \frac{43}{100} = .43 \qquad q' = \frac{54}{100} = .54$$

The u and u' are obtained from Table 5-4 in the same manner as for the u in biserial correlation. Thus:

For u: $.57 - .50 = .07$ From Table 5-4, $u = .393$

For u': $.54 - .50 = .04$ From Table 5-4, $u' = .397$

Substituting in the formula:

$$\sigma_{r_t} = \frac{\sqrt{(.57)(.43)(.46)(.54)}}{(.393)(.397)\sqrt{100}} = .16$$

From Table E, the t for df of 100 at the .01 level is 2.63. Therefore, the r_t necessary for significance at this level is: $.16 \times 2.63 = .421$. In the problem, the r_t of .656 is well beyond this amount, so the null hypothesis can be rejected with confidence.

As for biserial correlation, a t ratio may be obtained, as follows:

$$t = \frac{r_t}{\sigma_{r_t}} = \frac{.656}{.160} = 4.1$$

From Table E, last column, the t-ratio needed at the .01 level, as determined above, is 2.63. Thus, the significance of the r_t of .656 is beyond the .01 level.

DISCUSSION

Tetrachoric correlation is essentially equal to the product-moment correlation when the assumptions of continuity and linearity of regression are met. Continuous data may be dichotomized by dividing them into two categories at or near the median. In fact, the chinning and dipping scores in the illustrated problem were obtained in this manner. The correlations established by the two methods will not agree exactly, because the location of the scores are taken into account in the product-moment method, whereas only their presence in a quadrant (cell) is considered in the tetrachoric method.

However, the use of tetrachoric correlation should be avoided if possible, since its standard error is much larger than the standard error of the product-moment r; furthermore, σ_{r_t} differs for the various proportions of the dichotomies. Consider the problem above: The standard error of r_t at .00 is .16; for this same number of cases, the standard error of r at .00 is .10 $(1/\sqrt{N})$. To obtain a significant r at the .01 level: $.1 \times 2.60 = .26$; so, an r of .26 is significant at this level while the r_t must be .42. If the dichotomies had both been divided 50–50, the σ_{r_t} would be .15, which is the smallest amount possible for $N = 100$. The amount becomes larger as the dichotomies become widespread. As a consequence, at least twice as many subjects, and frequently more than twice as many, are needed to obtain the same standard error as for the product-moment method.

As for biserial correlation, transformation to the Fisher z coefficient is improper due to the instability of the standard error of r_t. This amount varies, as has been noted, with all proportions of the dichotomous variables. Furthermore, the amount of the standard error for this process is much greater than that for the product-moment r, a fact which indicates considerable instability in r_t itself.

Tetrachoric correlation should not be used when one of the cells contains no frequencies. Such a situation indicates curvilinearity in the data. Moreover, r_t should be avoided when the split in the dichotomies is very one-sided, such as 95–5, or even 90–10. In these situtaions, as has been pointed out, the standard error is very large.

Phi Coefficient

The phi coefficient was designed to correlate two dichotomous variables when both are point distributions. The concept of point distribution presented in the section on biserial correlation applies to the nature of these variables. The phi coefficient has a close relationship to chi square; as a consequence, chi square can be used to test its significance.

COMPUTATION

As for tetrachoric correlation a 2×2 table is constructed. The designations of the cells, rows, and columns are also the same: B and A for the upper cells, D and C for the lower cells, P and Q for totals of rows, and P' and Q' for totals of columns. The formula for computing phi coefficient (ϕ) is:

$$\phi = \frac{AD - BC}{\sqrt{PQP'Q'}} \qquad (5.11)$$

For an illustrated problem, hypothetical data of the eye color of fathers and sons are used. The distributions in the cells and the computation appear in Table 5-7. In this problem, $\phi = .54$.

TABLE 5-7
Phi Coefficient for
Eye Colors of Fathers and Sons

		Fathers' Eye Color		
		Brown	*Blue*	*Totals*
Sons' Eye Color	Blue	15 (B)	100 (A)	115 (P)
	Brown	55 (D)	30 (C)	85 (Q)
	Totals	70 (Q')	130 (P')	200

$$\phi = \frac{AD - BC}{\sqrt{PQP'Q'}}$$
$$= \frac{(100)(55) - (15)(30)}{\sqrt{(115)(85)(130)(70)}}$$
$$= .54$$

As indicated above, a convenient test of significance for ϕ is through chi square. The formula is:

$$\chi^2 = N\phi^2 \tag{5.12}$$

For this problem:

$$\chi^2 = (200)(.54^2)$$
$$= 58.32$$

Enter the chi-square table (Table G) with the usual degrees of freedom: $(r - 1)(c - 1) = (2 - 1)(2 - 1) = 1$. A chi square of 6.64 is necessary for significance at the .01 level. For this problem, therefore, the null hypothesis is rejected with considerable assurance, since the obtained chi square of 58.32 is much higher than the required amount.

An alternative method of computing the phi coefficient is to first compute chi square by the contingency-table method as described earlier in this chapter. The formula for phi coefficient is:

$$\phi = \sqrt{\frac{\chi^2}{N}} \tag{5.13}$$

LIMITATIONS

Typically, correlations vary from $+1.00$ to -1.00. This correlational range is also true of ϕ, but only when the dichotomies are evenly divided; when $P = Q$ and $P' = Q'$. When other proportions exist, the 2×2 table places restrictions upon ϕ which reduces its amount. If the investigator only wants to know whether the null hypothesis can be rejected, this situation does not present a problem. However, if he desires a coefficient comparable in magnitude to r, a correction must be made.

The correction of ϕ for the magnitude of r is accomplished by dividing the obtained ϕ by the maximum ϕ possible for the specific combinations of p and p'. This value is calculated from the following formula:

$$\phi_{max} = \sqrt{\frac{(p_j)(q_i)}{(q_j)(p_i)}} \tag{5.14}$$

in which: p_i = largest marginal proportion in the 2×2 table
$\qquad\quad p_j$ = highest marginal proportion for the other variable.
For the phi coefficient problem above, the largest marginal value is for P'. Thus, $p_i = 130/200 = .65$; then $q_i = 1 - p_i = .35$. The highest marginal value for the other variable is for P. Thus, $p_j = 115/200 = .58$; then $q_j =$

$1 - p_j = .42$. Substituting in formula 5.14:

$$\phi_{max} = \sqrt{\frac{(.58)(.35)}{(.42)(.63)}} = .86$$

Correcting ϕ for magnitude of r:

$$r_\phi = \frac{\phi}{\phi_{max}} = \frac{.54}{.86} = .63$$

ILLUSTRATED PROBLEM

The manner that phi coefficient may be used is illustrated in part of a study by Devine,[11] who investigated the relationships among the five components of a sociometric questionnaire (friends, movies, sports, homework, and party) for boys nine and eleven years of age. At each age, the choices of the boys for each pair of categories (2×2 table) were interrelated by use of the phi coefficient. The chi-square test was applied to determine the significance of these coefficients; and the phi coefficients were corrected for numerically equivalent product-moment correlations. The correlations between the categories were much higher for the 11-year-old boys than for the 9-year-old boys; consequently, all categories on the instrument were needed for peer status evaluation at nine years of age and should be considered separately when studying peer status. At age eleven years, only two categories (friends and homework) were necessary, since the other categories had high correlations with them.

Contingency Coefficient

The contingency coefficient provides a measure of correlation when each of the two variables is divided into two or more categories. Therefore, it can be used with 2×2 tables, but is not so restricted. However, as will be seen later, the tables should be square, i.e., both variables should have the same number of categories, such as 2×2, 3×3, 4×4, etc. This coefficient can be used with either parametric or nonparametric data.

The contingency coefficient (C) can be derived from chi square. Earlier in this chapter, the method of computing χ^2 from a contingency table was described, so this process will not be repeated here. Once χ^2 has been com-

[11] Barry M. Devine, "Analysis of Responses on a Sociometric Questionnaire and the Re-Examination of Structural and Strength Relationships for Nine and Eleven Year Old Boys," Microcard Master's Thesis, University of Oregon, 1960.

puted, C is obtained from the following formula:

$$C = \sqrt{\frac{\chi^2}{N + \chi^2}} \tag{5.15}$$

In the chi square problem involving the relation between the flavor and consumption of milk in the cafeteria (Table 5-1), χ^2 was 5.78. To compute C using formula 5.15:

$$C = \sqrt{\frac{5.78}{300 + 7.16}} = \sqrt{.019} = .104$$

As the χ^2 test for these data was not significant, neither is C, as χ^2 becomes the test of significance as was the case for the phi coefficient.

LIMITATIONS

The maximum size of C is limited by the number of categories into which the distributions is divided. Thus, magnitudes of C are only comparable when the number of cells in the comparisons is the same and none of these is comparable in magnitude to r. Therefore, it may be desirable to correct for the limitations imposed on C by contingency tables. Such a correction is available for square contingency tables only, which is the reason why both variables in such a problem should be confined to an equal number of categories. The formula for obtaining the maximum contingency coefficient is:

$$C_{max} = \sqrt{\frac{k - 1}{k}} \tag{5.16}$$

in which k is the number of rows or columns.

In data provided by J. Stuart Wickens, Groton Academy (Massachusetts), college men were given a posture test for kyphosis by two different methods: one method employed instrumentation and the other relied on subjective inspection. A 4×4 table was used; the contingency coefficient was .71. Computing C_{max} from formula 5.16:

$$C_{max} = \sqrt{\frac{4 - 1}{4}} = .866$$

Thus:

$$r_c = \frac{C}{C_{max}} = \frac{.71}{.866} = .82$$

In this problem, then, the correlation which is comparable in magnitude to the product-moment r is .82, rather than .71 (C).

ILLUSTRATED PROBLEM

Clarke and Stratton[12] investigated responses from a level of aspiration test based on maximum grip strength efforts applied to 110 nine-year-old boys. This test provided six scores, as follows: three aspiration discrepancies, computed as the difference between the subject's performance and aspiration scores; two performance differences, calculated as the difference between the subject's aspiration score and his immediately following performance score; and an aspiration adjustment discrepancy, given as the difference between the subject's two aspiration discrepancies. Each of these scores was divided into five groups based on grip strength scores, so that they could be used in computing contingency coefficients from 5 by 5 tables. The contingency coefficients were corrected for numerically equivalent product-moment correlations; in turn, these corrected contingency coefficients were converted to Fisher z coefficients and their differences tested for significance by application of the t ratio. Negative correlations were obtained between performance differences and aspiration discrepancies ranging between $-.517$ and $-.770$, when transformed to product-moment correlations. Intercorrelations of the three aspiration discrepancies were positive, between .606 to .759. It was suggested that in making specific recommendations for the grouping of subjects based on the magnitude of aspirations to achieve grip strength scores, three distinct groups may be identified: high-positive, low-positive to low-negative, and high-negative. The second aspiration appears to be the most meaningful of the discrepancy scores.

Curvilinear Relationships

In considering correlations throughout this book, the assumption of linearity of regression has been constantly made. Linearity was explained in Chapter 4 when regression lines were drawn on the correlational scattergram. The data followed a straight rather than a curved line; thus, a straight rather than a curved line was the line of best fit.

When, upon rare occasion, the regression line is curved, the product-moment coefficient is not proper to determine relationship; r calculated in such a situation will always be less than the true correlation. For example, consider the following pairs of scores for X and Y.

[12] H. Harrison Clarke and Stephen T. Stratton, "A Level of Aspiration Test Based on the Grip Strength Efforts of Nine-Year-Old Boys," *Child Development 33*, no. 4 (December 1962): 897–906.

X	Y
2	1
3	2
4	4
5	8
6	16

The X scores increased consistently by one point each time, while the Y scores doubled. The relationship is a perfect 1.00, but curved. The computed r is much less than 1.00.

The correlation ratio, or *eta* (η), should be used when the data are curvilinear. *Eta* will follow any line including a straight line; for linear data: $\eta = r$. However, two η's are always present, just as there are two regression lines; and, one line can be curvilinear and the other linear or both may be curvilinear. So, both may be computed, although only one of them may be of interest to the investigator, just as prediction in one direction only was shown to be frequently desired from the regression lines in Chapter 4.

The computation and interpretation of curvilinear relationships will not be presented here. Rather, the reader is referred to other statistics books if he should discover or suspect that his research data are curvilinear.

Other Nonparametric Statistics

At the beginning of this chapter, the nature of nonparametric statistics was explained. Occasionally throughout this text and the statistics chapters of the *Research Processes* book, such statistics have been presented, including median, percentiles, quartile deviation, rank-difference correlation, chi square, point-biserial correlation, phi coefficient, and contingency coefficient. Quite a number of other nonparametric statistics has been proposed to cover special situations encountered in educational research. The nature and use of several of these statistics will be mentioned here. For a detailed coverage of nonparametric statistics Siegel's book[13] is especially complete and useful.

SIGN TEST

The sign test is named from the fact that it uses plus and minus signs rather than quantitative data. The only assumption is that the data are continuous; no assumptions are made about the form of the distributions. The data must be available in pairs, as in correlation. The sign test consists of determining whether the scores in one set are above (+) or below (−) their

[13] Sidney Siegel, *Nonparametric Statistics for the Behavioral Sciences* (New York: McGraw-Hill Book Company, Inc., 1956).

corresponding scores in the other set. The null hypothesis is accepted if the differences between the number of signs is zero or the differences are too few as determined by a test of significance.

MEDIAN TEST

The median test determines the differences in central tendencies of two independent samples. The null hypothesis is that the two groups are from populations with the same median. For the computation, the two groups are combined and a single median is caluculated. If the two groups have been drawn at random from the same population, one-half of the scores in each group lie above and one-half lie below the common median. The observations are not paired or correlated and the N may differ in the two samples. The test of significance is through chi square.

MANN-WHITNEY U TEST

The Mann-Whitney U test is one of the most powerful of the nonparametric statistics. It is used to test the significance between two samples when the assumptions of the t test cannot be met. The null hypothesis is that the two samples have the same distribution. The null hypothesis is accepted if one-half of the scores in one sample are above scores in the other group and vice versa.

KOLMOGOROV-SMIRNOV TEST

The Kolmogorov-Smirnov test is a form of chi square for testing "goodness of fit" of an obtained frequency distribution to a hypothetical distribution. Differences between the K-S and the χ^2 tests are that the K-S test compares cumulative distributions and the comparison is made in terms of proportions rather than in terms of frequencies. The latter step arrives at a numerical value that is unaffected by sample size. The K-S test should be used rather than the χ^2 test when samples are small, which would require combining of adjacent categories before χ^2 could be properly computed. The K-S test is generally a more powerful test of significance than is χ^2.

The Kolmogorov-Smirnov two-sample test is an extension of the one-sample test, as it tests whether two independent samples have been drawn from the same population.

APPENDIX TABLES

TABLE A

F Ratios for Levels of Significance

Degrees of Freedom for Within Sets Variance	Degrees of Freedom for Between Sets Variance: 1	2	3	4	5	6
1	161.45*	199.50	215.72	224.57	230.17	233.97
	4052.10†	4999.03	5403.49	5625.14	5764.08	5859.39
2	18.51	19.00	19.16	19.25	19.30	19.33
	98.49	99.01	99.17	99.25	99.30	99.33
3	10.13	9.55	9.28	9.12	9.01	8.94
	34.12	30.81	29.46	28.71	28.24	27.91
4	7.71	6.94	6.59	6.39	6.26	6.16
	21.20	18.00	16.69	15.98	15.52	15.21
5	6.61	5.79	5.41	5.19	5.05	4.95
	16.26	13.27	12.06	11.39	10.97	10.67
6	5.99	5.14	4.76	4.53	4.39	4.28
	13.74	10.92	9.78	9.15	8.75	8.47
7	5.59	4.74	4.35	4.12	3.97	3.87
	12.25	9.55	8.45	7.85	7.46	7.19
8	5.32	4.46	4.07	3.84	3.69	3.58
	11.26	8.65	7.59	7.01	6.63	6.37
9	5.12	4.26	3.86	3.63	3.48	3.37
	10.56	8.02	6.99	6.42	6.06	5.80
10	4.96	4.10	3.71	3.48	3.33	3.22
	10.04	7.56	6.55	5.99	5.64	5.39
11	4.84	3.98	3.59	3.36	3.20	3.09
	9.65	7.20	6.22	5.67	5.32	5.07
12	4.75	3.88	3.49	3.26	3.11	3.00
	9.33	6.93	5.95	5.41	5.06	4.82
13	4.67	3.80	3.41	3.18	3.02	2.92
	9.07	6.70	5.74	5.20	4.86	4.62

* *Upper Figure: .05 Level*
† *Lower Figure: .01 Level*

Source: Table 18 in E. S. Pearson and H. O. Hartley, eds., Biometrika Tables for Statisticians, *vol. 1, 3rd ed. (Cambridge: Cambridge University Press, 1966); reprinted and abridged by permission of the editors and the trustees of* Biometrika.

Degrees of Freedom for Between Sets Variance

Degrees of Freedom for Within Sets Variance	1	2	3	4	5	6
14	4.60	3.74	3.34	3.11	2.96	2.85
	8.86	6.51	5.56	5.03	4.69	4.46
15	4.54	3.68	3.29	3.06	2.90	2.79
	8.68	6.36	5.42	4.89	4.56	4.32
16	4.49	3.63	3.24	3.01	2.85	2.74
	8.53	6.23	5.29	4.77	4.44	4.20
17	4.45	3.59	3.20	2.96	2.81	2.70
	8.40	6.11	5.18	4.67	4.34	4.10
18	4.41	3.55	3.16	2.93	2.77	2.66
	8.28	6.01	5.09	4.58	4.25	4.01
19	4.38	3.52	3.13	2.90	2.74	2.63
	8.18	5.93	5.01	4.50	4.17	3.94
20	4.35	3.49	3.10	2.87	2.71	2.60
	8.10	5.85	4.94	4.43	4.10	3.87
21	4.32	3.47	3.07	2.84	2.68	2.57
	8.02	5.78	4.87	4.37	4.04	3.81
22	4.30	3.44	3.05	2.82	2.66	2.55
	7.94	5.72	4.82	4.31	3.99	3.75
23	4.28	3.42	3.03	2.80	2.64	2.53
	7.88	5.66	4.76	4.26	3.94	3.71
24	4.26	3.40	3.01	2.78	2.62	2.51
	7.82	5.61	4.72	4.22	3.90	3.67
25	4.24	3.38	2.99	2.76	2.60	2.49
	7.77	5.57	4.68	4.18	3.86	3.63
26	4.22	3.37	2.98	2.74	2.59	2.47
	7.72	5.53	4.64	4.14	3.82	3.59
27	4.21	3.35	2.96	2.73	2.57	2.46
	7.68	5.49	4.60	4.11	3.78	3.56
28	4.20	3.34	2.95	2.71	2.56	2.44
	7.64	5.45	4.57	4.07	3.75	3.53
29	4.18	3.33	2.93	2.70	2.54	2.43
	7.60	5.42	4.54	4.04	3.73	3.50
30	4.17	3.32	2.92	2.69	2.53	2.42
	7.56	5.39	4.51	4.02	3.70	3.47
35	4.12	3.26	2.87	2.64	2.48	2.37
	7.42	5.27	4.40	3.91	3.59	3.37
40	4.08	3.23	2.84	2.61	2.45	2.34
	7.31	5.18	4.31	3.83	3.51	3.29
45	4.06	3.21	2.81	2.58	2.42	2.31
	7.23	5.11	4.25	3.77	3.45	3.23
50	4.03	3.18	2.79	2.56	2.40	2.29
	7.17	5.06	4.20	3.72	3.41	3.19
60	4.00	3.15	2.76	2.52	2.37	2.25
	7.08	4.98	4.13	3.65	3.34	3.12
70	3.98	3.13	2.74	2.50	2.35	2.23
	7.01	4.92	4.07	3.60	3.29	3.07
80	3.96	3.11	2.72	2.49	2.33	2.21
	6.96	4.88	4.04	3.56	3.26	3.04
90	3.95	3.10	2.71	2.47	2.32	2.20
	6.92	4.85	4.01	3.53	3.23	3.01
100	3.94	3.09	2.70	2.46	2.30	2.19
	6.90	4.82	3.98	3.51	3.21	2.99
125	3.92	3.07	2.68	2.44	2.29	2.17
	6.84	4.78	3.94	3.47	3.17	2.95

		1	2	3	4	5	6
				Degrees of Freedom for Between Sets Variance			
	150	3.90	3.06	2.66	2.43	2.27	2.16
		6.81	4.75	3.91	3.45	3.14	2.92
	200	3.89	3.04	2.65	2.42	2.26	2.14
		6.76	4.71	3.88	3.41	3.11	2.89
	300	3.87	3.03	2.64	2.41	2.25	2.13
		6.72	4.68	3.85	3.38	3.08	2.86
	400	3.86	3.02	2.63	2.40	2.24	2.12
		6.70	4.66	3.83	3.37	3.06	2.85
	500	3.86	3.01	2.62	2.39	2.23	2.11
		6.69	4.65	3.82	3.36	3.05	2.84
	1000	3.85	3.00	2.61	2.38	2.22	2.10
		6.66	4.63	3.80	3.34	3.04	2.82
	∞	3.84	2.99	2.60	2.37	2.21	2.09
		6.64	4.60	3.78	3.32	3.02	2.80

Degrees of Freedom for Within Sets Variance

TABLE B
Percentage Points of the Studentized Range

Error df	α	2	3	4	5	6	7	8	9	10	11
		\multicolumn{10}{c}{r = number of means or number of steps between ordered means}									
1	.05	17.97	26.98	38.82	37.08	40.41	43.12	45.40	47.36	49.07	50.59
	.01	90.03	135.0	164.3	185.6	202.2	215.8	227.2	237.0	245.6	253.2
2	.05	6.08	8.33	9.80	10.88	11.74	12.44	13.03	13.54	13.99	14.39
	.01	14.04	19.02	22.39	24.72	26.63	28.20	29.53	30.68	31.69	32.59
3	.05	4.50	5.91	6.82	7.50	8.04	8.48	8.85	9.18	9.46	9.72
	.01	8.26	10.62	12.17	13.33	14.24	15.00	15.64	16.20	16.69	17.13
4	.05	3.93	5.04	5.76	6.29	6.71	7.05	7.35	7.60	7.83	8.03
	.01	6.51	8.12	9.17	9.96	10.58	11.10	11.55	11.93	12.27	12.57
5	.05	3.64	4.60	5.22	5.67	6.03	6.33	6.58	6.80	6.99	7.17
	.01	5.70	6.98	7.80	8.42	8.91	9.32	9.67	9.97	10.24	10.48
6	.05	3.46	4.34	4.90	5.30	5.63	5.90	6.12	6.32	6.49	6.65
	.01	5.24	6.33	7.03	7.56	7.97	8.32	8.61	8.87	9.10	9.30
7	.05	3.34	4.16	4.68	5.06	5.36	5.61	5.82	6.00	6.16	6.30
	.01	4.95	5.92	6.54	7.01	7.37	7.68	7.94	8.17	8.37	8.55
8	.05	3.26	4.04	4.53	4.89	5.17	5.40	5.60	5.77	5.92	6.05
	.01	4.75	5.64	6.20	6.62	6.96	7.24	7.47	7.68	7.86	8.03
9	.05	3.20	3.95	4.41	4.76	5.02	5.24	5.43	5.59	5.74	5.87
	.01	4.60	5.43	5.96	6.35	6.66	6.91	7.13	7.33	7.49	7.65
10	.05	3.15	3.88	4.33	4.65	4.91	5.12	5.30	5.46	5.60	5.72
	.01	4.48	5.27	5.77	6.14	6.43	6.67	6.87	7.05	7.21	7.36
11	.05	3.11	3.82	4.26	4.57	4.82	5.03	5.20	5.35	5.49	5.61
	.01	4.39	5.15	5.62	5.97	6.25	6.48	6.67	6.84	6.99	7.13
12	.05	3.08	3.77	4.20	4.51	4.75	4.95	5.12	5.27	5.39	5.51
	.01	4.32	5.05	5.50	5.84	6.10	6.32	6.51	6.67	6.81	6.94
13	.05	3.06	3.73	4.15	4.45	4.69	4.88	5.05	5.19	5.32	5.43
	.01	4.26	4.96	5.40	5.73	5.98	6.19	6.37	6.53	6.67	6.79
14	.05	3.03	3.70	4.11	4.41	4.64	4.83	4.99	5.13	5.25	5.36
	.01	4.21	4.89	5.32	5.63	5.88	6.08	6.26	6.41	6.54	6.66
15	.05	3.01	3.67	4.08	4.37	4.59	4.78	4.94	5.08	5.20	5.31
	.01	4.17	4.84	5.25	5.56	5.80	5.99	6.16	6.31	6.44	6.55
16	.05	3.00	3.65	4.05	4.33	4.56	4.74	4.90	5.03	5.15	5.26
	.01	4.13	4.79	5.19	5.49	5.72	5.92	6.08	6.22	6.35	6.46
17	.05	2.98	3.63	4.02	4.30	4.52	4.70	4.86	4.99	5.11	5.21
	.01	4.10	4.74	5.14	5.43	5.66	5.85	6.01	6.15	6.27	6.38
18	.05	2.97	3.61	4.00	4.28	4.49	4.67	4.82	4.96	5.07	5.17
	.01	4.07	4.70	5.09	5.38	5.60	5.79	5.94	6.08	6.20	6.31
19	.05	2.96	3.59	3.98	4.25	4.47	4.65	4.79	4.92	5.04	5.14
	.01	4.05	4.67	5.05	5.33	5.55	5.73	5.89	6.02	6.14	6.25
20	.05	2.95	3.58	3.96	4.23	4.45	4.62	4.77	4.90	5.01	5.11
	.01	4.02	4.64	5.02	5.29	5.51	5.69	5.84	5.97	6.09	6.19
24	.05	2.92	3.53	3.90	4.17	4.37	4.54	4.68	4.81	4.92	5.01
	.01	3.96	4.55	4.91	5.17	5.37	5.54	5.69	5.81	5.92	6.02
30	.05	2.89	3.49	3.85	4.10	4.30	4.46	4.60	4.72	4.82	4.92
	.01	3.89	4.45	4.80	5.05	5.24	5.40	5.54	5.65	5.76	5.85
40	.05	2.86	3.44	3.79	4.04	4.23	4.39	4.52	4.63	4.73	4.82
	.01	3.82	4.37	4.70	4.93	5.11	5.26	5.39	5.50	5.60	5.69
60	.05	2.83	3.40	3.74	3.98	4.16	4.31	4.44	4.55	4.65	4.73
	.01	3.76	4.28	4.59	4.82	4.99	5.13	5.25	5.36	5.45	5.53
120	.05	2.80	3.36	3.68	3.92	4.10	4.24	4.36	4.47	4.56	4.64
	.01	3.70	4.20	4.50	4.71	4.87	5.01	5.12	5.21	5.30	5.37
∞	.05	2.77	3.31	3.63	3.86	4.03	4.17	4.29	4.39	4.47	4.55
	.01	3.64	4.12	4.40	4.60	4.76	4.88	4.99	5.08	5.16	5.23

Source: Table 29 in E. S. Pearson and H. O. Hartley, eds., Biometrika Tables for Statisticians, *vol. 1, 3rd ed. (Cambridge: Cambridge University Press, 1966); reprinted by permission of the editors and the trustees of* Biometrika.

TABLE C
Percentage Points of the Duncan New Multiple Range Test

Error df	Protection Level	\multicolumn{14}{c}{r = number of means for range being tested}													
		2	3	4	5	6	7	8	9	10	12	14	16	18	20
1	.05	18.00	18.00	18.00	18.00	18.00	18.00	18.00	18.00	18.00	18.00	18.00	18.00	18.00	18.00
	.01	90.00	90.00	90.00	90.00	90.00	90.00	90.00	90.00	90.00	90.00	90.00	90.00	90.00	90.00
2	.05	6.09	6.09	6.09	6.09	6.09	6.09	6.09	6.09	6.09	6.09	6.09	6.09	6.09	6.09
	.01	14.00	14.00	14.00	14.00	14.00	14.00	14.00	14.00	14.00	14.00	14.00	14.00	14.00	14.00
3	.05	4.50	4.50	4.50	4.50	4.50	4.50	4.50	4.50	4.50	4.50	4.50	4.50	4.50	4.50
	.01	8.26	8.50	8.60	8.70	8.80	8.90	8.90	9.00	9.00	9.00	9.10	9.20	9.30	9.30
4	.05	3.93	4.01	4.02	4.02	4.02	4.02	4.02	4.02	4.02	4.02	4.02	4.02	4.02	4.02
	.01	6.51	6.80	6.90	7.00	7.10	7.10	7.20	7.20	7.30	7.30	7.40	7.40	7.50	7.50
5	.05	3.64	3.74	3.79	3.83	3.83	3.83	3.83	3.83	3.83	3.83	3.83	3.83	3.83	3.83
	.01	5.70	5.96	6.11	6.18	6.26	6.33	6.40	6.44	6.50	6.60	6.60	6.70	6.70	6.80
6	.05	3.46	3.58	3.64	3.68	3.68	3.68	3.68	3.68	3.68	3.68	3.68	3.68	3.68	3.68
	.01	5.24	5.51	5.65	5.73	5.81	5.88	5.95	6.00	6.00	6.10	6.20	6.20	6.30	6.30
7	.05	3.35	3.47	3.54	3.58	3.60	3.61	3.61	3.61	3.61	3.61	3.61	3.61	3.61	3.61
	.01	4.95	5.22	5.37	5.45	5.53	5.61	5.69	5.73	5.80	5.80	5.90	5.90	6.00	6.00
8	.05	3.26	3.39	3.47	3.52	3.55	3.56	3.56	3.56	3.56	3.56	3.56	3.56	3.56	3.56
	.01	4.74	5.00	5.14	5.23	5.32	5.40	5.47	5.51	5.50	5.60	5.70	5.70	5.80	5.80
9	.05	3.20	3.34	3.41	3.47	3.50	3.52	3.52	3.52	3.52	3.52	3.52	3.52	3.52	3.52
	.01	4.60	4.86	4.99	5.08	5.17	5.25	5.32	5.36	5.40	5.50	5.50	5.60	5.70	5.70
10	.05	3.15	3.30	3.37	3.43	3.46	3.47	3.47	3.47	3.47	3.47	3.47	3.47	3.47	3.48
	.01	4.48	4.73	4.88	4.96	5.06	5.13	5.20	5.24	5.28	5.36	5.42	5.48	5.54	5.55
11	.05	3.11	3.27	3.35	3.39	3.43	3.44	3.45	3.46	3.46	3.46	3.46	3.46	3.47	3.48
	.01	4.39	4.63	4.77	4.86	4.94	5.01	5.06	5.12	5.15	5.24	5.28	5.34	5.38	5.39
12	.05	3.08	3.23	3.33	3.36	3.40	3.42	3.44	3.44	3.46	3.46	3.46	3.46	3.47	3.48
	.01	4.32	4.55	4.68	4.76	4.84	4.92	4.96	5.02	5.07	5.13	5.17	5.22	5.24	5.26
13	.05	3.06	3.21	3.30	3.35	3.38	3.41	3.42	3.44	3.45	3.45	3.46	3.46	3.47	3.47
	.01	4.26	4.48	4.62	4.69	4.74	4.84	4.88	4.94	4.98	5.04	5.08	5.13	5.14	5.15
14	.05	3.03	3.18	3.27	3.33	3.37	3.39	3.41	3.42	3.44	3.45	3.46	3.46	3.47	3.47
	.01	4.21	4.42	4.55	4.63	4.70	4.78	4.83	4.87	4.91	4.96	5.00	5.04	5.06	5.07

Table C. Continued

r = number of means for range being tested

Error df	Protection Level	2	3	4	5	6	7	8	9	10	12	14	16	18	20
15	.05	3.01	3.16	3.25	3.31	3.36	3.38	3.40	3.42	3.43	3.44	3.45	3.46	3.47	3.47
	.01	4.17	4.37	4.50	4.58	4.64	4.72	4.77	4.81	4.84	4.90	4.94	4.97	4.99	5.00
16	.05	3.00	3.15	3.23	3.30	3.34	3.37	3.39	3.41	3.43	3.44	3.45	3.46	3.47	3.47
	.01	4.13	4.34	4.45	4.54	4.60	4.67	4.72	4.76	4.79	4.84	4.88	4.91	4.93	4.94
17	.05	2.98	3.13	3.22	3.28	3.33	3.36	3.38	3.40	3.42	3.44	3.45	3.46	3.47	3.47
	.01	4.10	4.30	4.41	4.50	4.56	4.63	4.68	4.72	4.75	4.80	4.83	4.86	4.88	4.89
18	.05	2.97	3.12	3.21	3.27	3.32	3.35	3.37	3.39	3.41	3.43	3.45	3.46	3.47	3.47
	.01	4.07	4.27	4.38	4.46	4.53	4.59	4.64	4.68	4.71	4.76	4.79	4.82	4.84	4.85
19	.05	2.96	3.11	3.19	3.26	3.31	3.35	3.37	3.39	3.41	3.43	3.44	1.46	3.47	3.47
	.01	4.05	4.24	4.35	4.43	4.50	4.56	4.61	4.64	4.67	4.72	4.76	4.79	4.81	4.82
20	.05	2.95	3.10	3.18	3.25	3.30	3.34	3.36	3.38	3.40	3.43	3.44	3.46	3.46	3.47
	.01	4.02	4.22	4.33	4.40	4.47	4.53	4.58	4.61	4.65	4.69	4.73	4.76	4.78	4.79
22	.05	2.93	3.08	3.17	3.24	3.29	3.32	3.35	3.37	3.39	3.42	3.44	3.45	3.46	3.47
	.01	3.99	4.17	4.28	4.36	4.42	4.48	4.53	4.57	4.60	4.65	4.68	4.71	4.74	4.75
24	.05	2.92	3.07	3.15	3.22	3.28	3.31	3.34	3.37	3.38	3.41	3.44	3.45	3.46	3.47
	.01	3.96	4.14	4.24	4.33	4.39	4.44	4.49	4.53	4.57	4.62	4.64	4.67	4.70	4.72
26	.05	2.91	3.06	3.14	3.21	3.27	3.30	3.34	3.36	3.38	3.41	3.43	3.45	3.46	3.47
	.01	3.93	4.11	4.21	4.30	4.36	4.41	4.46	4.50	4.53	4.58	4.62	4.65	4.67	4.69
28	.05	2.90	3.04	3.13	3.20	3.26	3.30	3.33	3.35	3.37	3.40	3.43	3.45	3.46	3.47
	.01	3.91	4.08	4.18	4.28	4.34	4.39	4.43	4.47	4.51	4.56	4.60	4.62	4.65	4.67
30	.05	2.89	3.04	3.12	3.20	3.25	3.29	3.32	3.35	3.37	3.40	3.43	3.44	3.46	3.47
	.01	3.89	4.06	4.16	4.22	4.32	4.36	4.41	4.45	4.48	4.54	4.58	4.61	4.63	4.65
40	.05	2.86	3.01	3.10	3.17	3.22	3.27	3.30	3.33	3.35	3.39	3.42	3.44	3.46	3.47
	.01	3.82	3.99	4.10	4.17	4.24	4.30	4.34	4.37	4.41	4.46	4.51	4.54	4.57	4.59
60	.05	2.83	2.98	3.08	3.14	3.20	3.24	3.28	3.31	3.33	3.37	3.40	3.43	3.45	3.47
	.01	3.76	3.92	4.03	4.12	4.17	4.23	4.27	4.31	4.34	4.39	4.44	4.47	4.50	4.53
100	.05	2.80	2.95	3.05	3.12	3.18	3.22	3.26	3.29	3.32	3.36	3.40	3.42	3.45	3.47
	.01	3.71	3.86	3.93	4.06	4.11	4.17	4.21	4.25	4.29	4.35	4.38	4.42	4.45	4.48
∞	.05	2.77	2.92	3.02	3.09	3.15	3.19	3.23	3.26	3.29	3.34	3.38	3.41	3.44	3.47
	.01	3.64	3.80	3.90	3.98	4.04	4.09	4.14	4.17	4.20	4.26	4.31	4.34	4.38	4.41

Source: Biometrics, vol. 11 (1955): 1–42; reprinted by permission of David B. Duncan and the editor of Biometrics.

r	$\sqrt{1 - r^2}$	r	$\sqrt{1 - r^2}$	r	$\sqrt{1 - r^2}$
.00	1.0000	.34	.9404	.68	.7332
.01	.9999	.35	.9367	.69	.7238
.02	.9998	.36	.9330	.70	.7141
.03	.9995	.37	.9290	.71	.7042
.04	.9992	.38	.9250	.72	.6940
.05	.9987	.39	.9208	.73	.6834
.06	.9982	.40	.9165	.74	.6726
.07	.9975	.41	.9121	.75	.6614
.08	.9968	.42	.9075	.76	.6499
.09	.9959	.43	.9028	.77	.6380
.10	.9950	.44	.8980	.78	.6258
.11	.9939	.45	.8930	.79	.6131
.12	.9928	.46	.8879	.80	.6000
.13	.9915	.47	.8827	.81	.5864
.14	.9902	.48	.8773	.82	.5724
.15	.9887	.49	.8717	.83	.5578
.16	.9871	.50	.8660	.84	.5426
.17	.9854	.51	.8617	.85	.5268
.18	.9837	.52	.8542	.86	.5103
.19	.9818	.53	.8480	.87	.4931
.20	.9798	.54	.8417	.88	.4750
.21	.9777	.55	.8352	.89	.4560
.22	.9755	.56	.8285	.90	.4359
.23	.9732	.57	.8216	.91	.4146
.24	.9708	.58	.8146	.92	.3919
.25	.9682	.59	.8074	.93	.3676
.26	.9656	.60	.8000	.94	.3412
.27	.9629	.61	.7924	.95	.3122
.28	.9600	.62	.7846	.96	.2800
.29	.9570	.63	.7766	.97	.2431
.30	.9539	.64	.7684	.98	.1990
.31	.9507	.65	.7599	.99	.1411
.32	.9474	.66	.7513	1.00	.0000
.33	.9440	.67	.7424		

TABLE E
Correlation Coefficients and t Ratios
Significant at the .05 (Upper) and .01 (Lower) Levels

Degrees of Freedom	Number of Variables						
	2	3	4	5	6	7	t
1	.997	.999	.999	.999	1.000	1.000	12.706
	1.000	1.000	1.000	1.000	1.000	1.000	63.657
2	.950	.975	.983	.987	.990	.992	4.303
	.990	.995	.997	.998	.998	.998	9.925
3	.878	.930	.950	.961	.968	.973	3.182
	.959	.976	.983	.987	.990	.991	5.841
4	.811	.881	.912	.930	.942	.950	2.776
	.917	.949	.962	.970	.975	.979	4.604
5	.754	.836	.874	.898	.914	.925	2.571
	.874	.917	.937	.949	.957	.963	4.032
6	.707	.795	.839	.867	.886	.900	2.447
	.834	.886	.911	.927	.938	.946	3.707
7	.666	.758	.807	.838	.860	.876	2.365
	.798	.855	.885	.904	.918	.928	3.499
8	.632	.726	.777	.811	.835	.854	2.306
	.765	.827	.860	.882	.898	.909	3.355
9	.602	.697	.750	.786	.812	.832	2.262
	.735	.800	.836	.861	.878	.891	3.250
10	.576	.671	.726	.763	.790	.812	2.228
	.708	.776	.814	.840	.859	.874	3.169
11	.553	.648	.703	.741	.770	.792	2.201
	.684	.753	.793	.821	.841	.857	3.106
12	.532	.627	.683	.722	.751	.774	2.179
	.661	.732	.773	.802	.824	.841	3.055
13	.514	.608	.664	.703	.733	.757	2.160
	.641	.712	.755	.785	.807	.825	3.012
14	.497	.590	.646	.686	.717	.741	2.145
	.623	.694	.737	.768	.792	.810	2.977
15	.482	.574	.630	.670	.701	.726	2.131
	.606	.677	.721	.752	.776	.796	2.947
16	.468	.559	.615	.655	.686	.712	2.120
	.590	.662	.706	.738	.762	.782	2.921
17	.456	.545	.601	.641	.673	.698	2.110
	.575	.647	.691	.724	.749	.769	2.898
18	.444	.532	.587	.628	.660	.686	2.101
	.561	.633	.678	.710	.736	.756	2.878
19	.433	.520	.575	.615	.647	.674	2.093
	.549	.620	.665	.698	.723	.744	2.861
20	.423	.509	.563	.604	.636	.662	2.086
	.537	.608	.652	.685	.712	.733	2.845
21	.413	.498	.552	.592	.624	.651	2.080
	.526	.596	.641	.674	.700	.722	2.831
22	.404	.488	.542	.582	.614	.640	2.074
	.515	.585	.630	.663	.690	.712	2.819
23	.396	.479	.532	.572	.604	.630	2.069
	.505	.574	.619	.652	.679	.701	2.807
24	.388	.470	.523	.562	.594	.621	2.064
	.496	.565	.609	.642	.669	.692	2.797

Number of Variables

Degrees of Freedom	2	3	4	5	6	7	t
25	.381	.462	.514	.553	.585	.612	2.060
	.487	.555	.600	.633	.660	.682	2.787
26	.374	.454	.506	.545	.576	.603	2.056
	.478	.546	.590	.624	.651	.673	2.779
27	.367	.446	.498	.536	.568	.594	2.052
	.470	.538	.582	.615	.642	.664	2.771
28	.361	.439	.490	.529	.560	.586	2.048
	.463	.530	.573	.606	.634	.656	2.763
29	.355	.432	.482	.521	.552	.579	2.045
	.456	.522	.565	.598	.625	.648	2.756
30	.349	.426	.476	.514	.545	.571	2.042
	.449	.514	.558	.591	.618	.640	2.750
35	.325	.397	.445	.482	.512	.538	2.030
	.418	.481	.523	.556	.582	.605	2.724
40	.304	.373	.419	.455	.484	.509	2.021
	.393	.454	.494	.526	.552	.575	2.704
45	.288	.353	.397	.432	.460	.485	2.014
	.372	.430	.470	.501	.527	.549	2.690
50	.273	.336	.379	.412	.440	.464	2.008
	.354	.410	.449	.479	.504	.526	2.678
60	.250	.308	.348	.380	.406	.429	2.000
	.325	.377	.414	.442	.466	.488	2.660
70	.233	.286	.324	.354	.379	.401	1.994
	.302	.351	.386	.413	.436	.456	2.648
80	.217	.269	.304	.332	.356	.377	1.990
	.283	.330	.362	.389	.411	.431	2.638
90	.205	.254	.288	.315	.338	.358	1.987
	.267	.312	.343	.368	.390	.409	2.632
100	.195	.241	.274	.300	.322	.341	1.984
	.254	.297	.327	.351	.372	.390	2.626
125	.174	.216	.246	.269	.290	.307	1.979
	.228	.266	.294	.316	.335	.352	2.616
150	.159	.198	.225	.247	.266	.282	1.976
	.208	.244	.270	.290	.308	.324	2.609
200	.138	.172	.196	.215	.231	.246	1.972
	.181	.212	.234	.253	.269	.283	2.601
300	.113	.141	.160	.176	.190	.202	1.968
	.148	.174	.192	.208	.221	.233	2.592
400	.098	.122	.139	.153	.165	.176	1.966
	.128	.151	.167	.180	.192	.202	2.588
500	.088	.109	.124	.137	.148	.157	1.965
	.115	.135	.150	.162	.172	.182	2.586
1,000	.062	.077	.088	.097	.105	.112	1.962
	.081	.096	.106	.115	.122	.129	2.581
∞							1.960
							2.576

Reprinted by permission from Correlation and Machine Calculation *by H. A. Wallace and G. W. Snedecor, © 1931 by Iowa State College Press, Ames, Iowa.*

Conversion of Product-Moment Correlation to Fisher's z Coefficient Equivalent*

r	z	r	z	r	z	r	z	r	z	r	z
.25	.26	.40	.42	.55	.62	.70	.87	.85	1.26	.950	1.83
.26	.27	.41	.44	.56	.63	.71	.89	.86	1.29	.955	1.89
.27	.28	.42	.45	.57	.65	.72	.91	.87	1.33	.960	1.95
.28	.29	.43	.46	.58	.66	.73	.93	.88	1.38	.965	2.01
.29	.30	.44	.47	.59	.68	.74	.95	.89	1.42	.970	2.09
.30	.31	.45	.48	.60	.69	.75	.97	.90	1.47	.975	2.18
.31	.32	.46	.50	.61	.71	.76	1.00	.905	1.50	.980	2.30
.32	.33	.47	.51	.62	.73	.77	1.02	.910	1.53	.985	2.44
.33	.34	.48	.52	.63	.74	.78	1.05	.915	1.56	.990	2.65
.34	.35	.49	.54	.64	.76	.79	1.07	.920	1.59	.995	2.99
.35	.37	.50	.55	.65	.78	.80	1.10	.925	1.62		
.36	.38	.51	.56	.66	.79	.81	1.13	.930	1.66		
.37	.39	.52	.58	.67	.81	.82	1.16	.935	1.70		
.38	.40	.53	.59	.68	.83	.83	1.19	.940	1.74		
.39	.41	.54	.60	.69	.85	.84	1.22	.945	1.78		

* r's under .25 may be taken as equivalent to z's.

df	0.20	0.10	0.05	0.02	0.01
1	1.642	2.706	3.841	5.412	6.635
2	3.219	4.605	5.991	7.824	9.210
3	4.642	6.251	7.815	9.837	11.345
4	5.989	7.779	9.488	11.668	13.277
5	7.289	9.236	11.071	13.388	15.086
6	8.558	10.645	12.592	15.033	16.812
7	9.803	12.017	14.067	16.622	18.475
8	11.030	13.362	15.507	18.168	20.090
9	12.242	14.684	16.919	19.679	21.666
10	13.442	15.987	18.307	21.161	23.209
11	14.631	17.275	19.675	22.618	24.725
12	15.812	18.549	21.026	24.054	26.217
13	16.985	19.812	22.362	25.472	27.688
14	18.151	21.064	23.685	26.873	29.141
15	19.311	22.307	24.996	28.259	30.578
16	20.465	23.542	26.296	29.633	32.000
17	21.615	24.769	27.587	30.995	33.409
18	22.760	25.989	28.869	32.346	34.805
19	23.900	27.204	30.144	33.687	36.191
20	25.038	28.412	31.410	35.020	37.566
21	26.171	29.615	32.671	36.343	38.932
22	27.301	30.813	33.924	37.659	40.289
23	28.429	32.007	35.172	38.968	41.638
24	29.553	33.196	36.415	40.270	42.980
25	30.675	34.382	37.652	41.566	44.314
26	31.795	35.563	38.885	42.856	45.642
27	32.912	36.741	40.113	44.140	46.963
28	34.027	37.916	41.337	45.419	48.278
29	35.139	39.087	42.557	46.693	49.588
30	36.250	40.256	43.773	47.962	50.892

Source: Table 8 in E. S. Pearson and H. O. Hartley, eds., Biometrika Tables for Statisticians, *vol. 1, 3rd ed. (Cambridge: Cambridge University Press, 1966); reprinted and abridged by permission of the editors and the trustees of* Biometrika.

INDEX